To Walk Among the Gods

By Eugene Coco MD

ISBN:
Print Version 978-1-7367599-2-9
E-pub Version 978-1-7367599-3-6

Printed in the United States of America

The characters in this tale are fictional, but the cases are true, as true as I can remember them, and as true as I can write them.

To the exceptional men and women of the medical profession who are called to relieve suffering, prevent disability, and prolong life. May they all walk among the gods someday.

To my muse, my collaborator, the light of my life, and to her future, Claire.

Table of Contents

Chapter 1

Orientation

"Most especially must I tread with care in matters of life
and death. If it is given to me to save a life, all thanks.
But it may also be within my power to take a life; this awesome
responsibility must be faced with great humbleness and
awareness of my own frailty, above all, I must not play God."
Hippocratic Oath

When Apollo's son, Asclepius, the first physician, became so skilled at healing he could bring the dead back to life, Zeus slew him with a thunderbolt because he was afraid Asclepius might render all mankind immortal. But because of his ability to heal, Asclepius became a hero to the people, so Zeus raised him up to Olympus to walk among the gods.

Dave Cameron was a naïve, idealistic young man who dreamed of becoming a physician. He never considered doing anything else with his life. To realize his dream and join Asclepius in the ranks of those privileged to walk among the gods, he first had to gain the skills needed to grapple with death. To gain those skills, he would have to travel a daunting, demanding, difficult road. His journey on that road began the day he walked out of the sticky humid white-hot heat of the Southern summer sun into the cool conditioned air of the waiting area of the administrative offices of University Hospital.

Among the diverse group of young men and women nervously milling around in the cramped room Dave immediately recognized two of his former roommates. Henry was Dave's roommate in college. He

1

was wealthy with significant yearly income from a trust fund, plus additional revenue from his family's oil holdings. His manner of speaking, the way he carried himself, and his clothes gave him an unmistakable golden aura. He never attended a public school, spent a year of prep school at a posh academy in Italy, and did a semester of college at the Sorbonne in Paris. But Henry did not manifest the over privileged, elitist attitude that infected most members of his socio-economic class. He was a scientist: logical, rational, and overly pragmatic. "Do you have a place to live yet, Dave? If you don't, we have a room open at the house where I live. It's an old Victorian, we each have a large bedroom with a sitting area, a connecting bathroom, and there's plenty of extra living space."

"I rented a one-bedroom apartment on the North Side in a singles complex with a pool, but what about you, Mike?" Mike did not answer immediately because he was distracted by Henry's gold Rolex watch, custom tailored attire, and expensive Italian shoes. Dave was accustomed to Henry's displays of wealth, but Mike was momentarily speechless.

Finally, he answered, "I'm staying in a Motel 6 trying to find a place." Mike was Dave's roommate during his clerkship in medical school. He grew up in a working-class neighborhood, was the first in his family to attend college, and now he had graduated from medical school. He used his intelligence to leave his blue-collar background behind, but in the process, he became exceedingly competitive and was known as a "gunner" in school: someone who climbs over the backs of their classmates, shooting them down in order to improve their own class ranking. His confidence produced a cockiness in his manner, his achievements infused his demeanor with arrogance, and he was an unabashed self-promoter.

"There's a party at our house tomorrow night, Mike; a kind of 'last rites' celebration for those of us starting our internship. Come to the party, meet the other two guys, and check it out. Dave, I want you to come to the party and meet one of the flight attendants who lives next door. She was dating Bar, but he's gone now. That's why we have a room open, he left for Boston to do his internship in a Harvard program."

"Why are you introducing me to this flight attendant?" Dave knew Henry ignored anything that did not concern him directly, so he was surprised by the offer to introduce him to a woman.

"I'm dating someone." Henry only dated women who came from money, and he was very particular about the men he associated with, always evaluating them carefully to make sure they were genuine. He was a target because of his wealth.

Dave continued to be puzzled by Henry's uncharacteristic behavior. "This is not like you, Henry, getting involved and setting someone up."

"I'm not setting you up, I'm simply facilitating a meeting between two people I like, but wait until you meet her. A lot of men are after her since she dumped Bar, but I think you two will connect." Henry continued to praise Sharon's qualities to Dave, so he began to get excited about meeting her. Eventually all the new interns were registered, and orientation was ready to begin.

Walking to the main conference room, Henry told Dave his plans, "I don't want to practice medicine in a commercial healthcare system. I don't want to be concerned about patient retention and satisfaction or be forced to use a computer-generated algorithm of 'best practice' guidelines. The last thing I want is to be constrained by the gate keeping actions of some insurance administrator. I'm going to apply for a fellowship in infectious disease and do research. I don't want to teach either. Medical schools are businesses too, and to teach I would have to deal with the politics of the institution's financial viability. I want to do pure research and avoid any contact with the current healthcare model that's controlled by the private sector." They reached the conference room and found seats.

The hospital administrator welcomed them with a short speech. The director of nursing talked about the need to interact with the nursing staff in a professional manner and gave them guidelines for working with student nurses. The head dietitian was next on the agenda. "Your meals are free if you are in the hospital. Everyone gets breakfast and lunch, and you get dinner if you are on call or working late." Then she talked about the role of dietitians on the wards. The last speaker was the head of the laundry. He told them their lab coats and OR shoes would be in the laundry on Monday in packages labeled with their names. "Make sure you turn in your coat and shoe sizes before you leave here today. You can wear scrubs in the ED, L and D, the Nursery, surgery, and if you are on call." After the presentations, the administrator dismissed them and instructed them to report to the conference room of their service.

Mike and Henry were straight medicine interns and Dave's first rotation was medicine. When they reached the conference room, Doctor Sheffield, an icon of medical education, was standing beside the door dressed in a gray suit next to a nice looking, well-groomed young man in a lab coat. His Department of Medicine at the medical school had produced two Nobel Laureates and his postgraduate training program had produced two more. "Come in and take a seat. I want to welcome you. I'm Doctor Sheffield, and this is Doctor Jeffrey, the chief resident. Doctor Jeffery is going to pass out packets that include your schedules and team assignments. He will go over all that information with you, then take you on a tour of the hospital. When the tour is finished, you are free to go, but report back to your ward or the ED by ten Tuesday morning to start taking over from the outgoing teams."

Doctor Sheffield centered himself at the front of the room. He was tall, lean, and angular with thick, long gray hair, and piercing gray eyes. He looked at the new interns the way Moses must have looked at the Israelites when he came down from the mountain with the ten commandments. "Doctors: that is what you are now, doctors. You have been granted that title along with the great privilege of spending your life as a physician. You earned the title with four years of college, four years of medical school, countless hours of study, and hard work. Now you are one of us; you are a doctor, and you will spend the rest of your life in one of the most rewarding, fulfilling, and satisfying callings one can have. Make no mistake about it: it is a calling. If you are not called to be a physician, you do not belong here, and you should get up and leave right now. If you are here because you want a good income, because your father or mother is a doctor, because your parents or grandparents want you to be a doctor, because you want the profession to benefit you in some way, or because it just seemed like a good idea, you should get up and leave right now because you do not belong here. But if you are called to serve humanity, if you are driven and compelled to relieve suffering, prevent disability, and prolong life in your fellow human beings, then welcome to University Hospital and the Department of Medicine.

"I want you to describe yourself in one sentence. Who are you, what is your philosophy of life, everything about you in one sentence? Go ahead, I will give you a little time." Sheffield paused. "Go over the sentence in your mind. If you did not begin the sentence with, 'I am a doctor,' you need to reevaluate who you are because being a physician needs to define you. What does that mean? It means you relieve the suffering, prevent the disability, and prolong the life of your patients, or all humankind if you do research or teach. What higher calling can there be? This next year will prepare you to do that, but make no mistake, it will challenge you to your very core. You will suffer from lack of sleep. The stress will be overwhelming, and the demands will be beyond what you think you can endure, but when you finish your internship here, you will be well trained, and ready to be a physician. Thank you for your time. Doctor Jeffrey, they are all yours."

Doctor Jeffrey had the look and mannerisms of a face man who occupied a high-profile visible position. "Doctors, check your team assignments. Ward teams consist of two interns, a junior resident, and senior resident. There are four ED teams with two interns and a junior resident on each team with a senior resident assigned to oversee two teams. Call is every third night on the wards, rotating from Team One to Team Three, so Team One is on call on July first. In the ED, Teams One and Two rotate with Teams Three and Four, with the teams alternating between Major Medicine and Minor Medicine. Major Medicine goes from seven AM to seven AM. Minor Medicine goes from seven AM until seven PM with everyone out of Minor Medicine by nine PM. Teams in the ED are not expected to attend any conferences or to meet with staff, instead they are expected to always be available in the ED. On the wards, rounds start at seven AM, and you meet with your attending at ten AM. Rounds with the chief are at eleven and the team on call the day before will have their charts ready. Lunch is at twelve with the clinic starting at one PM and ending at five. Follow-up rounds are at five PM, and you should be out of the hospital by seven."

The chief resident looked around for questions: there were none. "There are seven holidays. Only the teams on call and working the ED that day have to come in. The team on call will round for the other teams, and there will be no meetings or conferences. If the holiday is on a Saturday, the team on Sunday will round for everyone, so they are the only ones who come in on the day after the holiday. Grand rounds are on Saturday at eleven AM; attendance is not mandatory but encouraged. Rounds on Saturday and Sunday are at eight AM and there are no meetings or conferences on Sunday. You get one week of vacation. You will average eighty to a hundred hours a week in the hospital, so get ready to put your social life on hold. Are there any questions?" Again, there were no questions.

They finished the hospital tour and Jeffery dismissed them, "Monday you need to turn in your paperwork, pick up your OR shoes and lab coats, and get your parking permits. After that you are free until Tuesday morning."

"How about a beer?" Mike liked to take charge. Henry directed them to an Irish pub he knew, they found a table, and ordered three Guinness drafts. "I checked the schedules and we're all off on the Fourth, so maybe we can do something together." He had already decided to take the room at Henry's house, because he was sure he would benefit from being one of his roommates.

"I'll talk to Sherry about organizing a picnic in the park. We will have a picnic, listen to the concert, watch the fireworks, and have a party afterwards. I'll ask Connie to look for a date for you, Mike." Mike finished his beer and left, but Henry and Dave continued to talk. "He seems OK, but I'm not sure. He's pretty rough around the edges."

"I was rough around the edges when we met."

"You weren't rough around the edges. You were a diamond in the rough. All you needed was a little polishing. I'm not sure this guy is a gemstone, much less a diamond." They parted after exchanging addresses and phone numbers, with Dave promising to be at the party tomorrow night.

Driving to his apartment, Dave reflected on how Henry had "polished" him. Henry taught him how to dress well, about food, wine, and art. Henry had indeed polished him by elevating his level of sophistication and basically giving him a one-on-one liberal arts education.

Dave woke up the next morning fantasizing about the woman he was going to meet that night. He had a country cousin he grew up with and they had remained close. She once told him, "I hope you don't fly over all the flowers in the garden and land on a pile of manure in the barnyard." He had certainly flitted over a flower or two, and he had been in the barnyard a couple of times, but no matter how good or bad his previous relationships had been, none of them had been what he wanted. He wanted an all-consuming, unconditional love like the ones he read about in the novels he enjoyed. He might be too idealistic, but that is what he wanted and that's who he was: a naïve, romantic guy looking forward to the girl he was going to meet.

Later, he called Henry. "Can you meet me for lunch? I want to talk to you about some things."

"I'll meet you at the Irish pub." Henry was sitting in a back booth waiting for him when he arrived. "What did you want to talk about?"

"I want to talk about the broken bodies and devastating diseases we deal with. I want to talk about the pathos we encounter treating patients. I want to talk about the blood, vomit, pus, body fluids, and smells we're exposed to. I can't deal with the smells. I want to talk about being responsible, not just watching someone else make the decisions. I'm not sure I can deal with the on-the-job training we have to do." Dave had been struggling with insecurities about his chosen profession since his clerkship in medical school, and it felt good to finally open up to someone about them.

"I hear you about the smells. I barfed in front of my entire surgery team. The nurses laughed at me, made jokes at my expense, and gave me a nickname I'll never divulge. But I couldn't help it, the smell hit me, and the barf came out of me." Henry's face soured briefly, then returned to his normal calm expression. "You have to focus on the case and shut everything else out. Don't think about anything but the diagnosis and treatment. Keep it scientific and outcome driven."

"You're talking about depersonalizing the patients. They aren't real people with real names; they're the CHF patient, the diabetic, the GI bleed. I know you can't do the job if you get emotionally involved, but I have trouble ignoring the humanity of it."

"I understand. I drink more to deal with it. Detached sociopaths like Bar seem to thrive. Empathy is good, but it's a double-edged sword that cuts both ways. If you don't manage your emotions, they can turn on you."

"I'm sorry, but I needed to talk to someone. I'm not sure I can do this, and what's more, I'm not sure I want to do it. That's a hell of a thing to discover at this stage of the game."

"Believe in yourself, Dave. I know that sounds like a cliché to patronize you, but it's true. You're smart and you're tough. You can do this, and I know you want to do it. Like Sheffield said, you're called. I'm sorry I'm not more helpful, but it's really up to you."

After lunch, Dave drove to his apartment, took a swim, and spent the rest of the afternoon relaxing in a lounge chair thinking about what Henry said. As a student, he had seen some very disturbing things, and no matter how detached he tried to be, he couldn't help being affected. *I have to find ways to insulate myself from the emotional onslaught of a place like University Hospital and I have to find ways to cope with the personal tragedies I encounter there? I will be the one responsible; responsible for another person's life. That's a crushing responsibility.*

Later he showered, shaved, doused himself with cologne, put on his lucky T-shirt, his favorite jeans, and followed Henry's directions to the house on the park. It was a large old Victorian with a similar house next to it and looked as if the same builder had built both of them. The front door was open, and he could hear people talking, so he walked in.

The house had the distinct feel of the bygone era. The rooms had lofty ceilings with wainscoting, hardwood floors, and thick plaster walls. The entry way led to a hall that ended in a staircase with a landing at the top. There was an opening on the left to a large dining room. A pony keg with red plastic cups was at one end of a big table and bottles of wine with plastic wine glasses were at the other end. The opening on the right led to another larger room furnished with mismatched couches and chairs, plus the ever-present card table found in all male-dominated communal living quarters.

Henry was sitting on one of the couches between two women. The one on his right was a small woman dressed in an expensive work casual outfit and everything about her was prim and proper from her perfectly coiffed hair to her stylish shoes. The one on his left was looking at Henry, so he only saw her in a partial profile at first. She was a classic beauty with balanced features, an alluring mouth, and long soft auburn hair with highlights. She was dressed in a close-fitting white blouse with the top buttons left unbuttoned to expose a glimpse of the swell of her full, firm breasts, and a short black skirt that drew attention to her long, slim perfectly shaped legs. She was dressed to accentuate their best features, and she had that stylistic flair of a European woman. If she had been wearing a scarf, he would have been certain she was French.

She turned to look at him, and her unusual eyes met his eyes in an unwavering gaze. They were sensual and almost colorless. They elevated her beauty to another level and made her look like a mystical ethereal being from another world. He smiled to try to cover his astonishment and she returned his smile with a slight hint of mirth at the corners of her mouth, then she looked him up and down. He heard women talk about guys undressing them with their eyes and now he knew what they meant. She evaluated him from head to foot with a penetrating stare that made him feel completely exposed, not just physically, but as if she could see into his very essence with her remarkable eyes. He regained his composure and broadened his smile into a grin. *Don't just stand here grinning like an idiot, you idiot. That's an unbelievably beautiful woman and she is here to meet you. Get your act together and do something or say something before she realizes you are an idiot.* He started walking toward her and that's when Henry saw him and stood up. "Dave."

The ethereal being stood up too and Dave saw just how striking she was. She was tall, lithe, and graceful. It occurred to him that was why she stood up, not to be introduced to him, but so he could see how stunning she was. Henry turned to the woman on his right, "Sherry, this is Dave, my college roommate. Dave, this is Sherry." She extended a limp hand, and he took it gently to acknowledge her. Henry turned to the beauty on his left, "And this is Sharon Kelly, a flight attendant who lives next door, Sharon, this is Doctor David Cameron." She did not extend her hand but just stood there to let him take her in.

"Sherry, move over a little so Dave can squeeze in beside Sharon." They sat down, and she turned to face him. Her makeup drew attention to her translucent eyes. They had emerald green rings around the edges of irises that were so pale they were almost white. Once she fixed his gaze with her other worldly eyes, she knew he was hooked. The only question was whether she should reel him in and keep him, or throw him back. Dave was completely aware of where things stood after that look.

"Dave, you need a beer. There is beer in the dining room." Henry pointed to the opening across the hall.

"I need something too." Sharon stood up and led him to the dining room. At the table, he asked her what she wanted. "A beer is fine."

"I didn't take you for a beer girl." He took two red cups, pulled two beers from the keg, and handed one to her.

Their eyes met again as she looked at him over the rim of her beer cup. "Normally you would be right, but I can nurse a beer along a lot longer at a party than a glass of wine. Do you want to go back to talk to Henry and Sherry?"

He was transfixed by her eyes, but managed an answer. "No. I've heard everything Henry has to say, and he's heard everything I have to say."

She laughed. "What about your other friend? Isn't he coming tonight? He may be here already. Do you want to go back and check?"

He knew it was a critical moment. If they went back, she was throwing him back. If she stayed and talked to him, he still had a chance with her. He didn't want to be rejected by the most desirable woman he had ever met, so he made his move. "Henry introduced us because he thought we had a lot in common. Normally he doesn't get involved and do that sort of thing. I think we should trust him and see what happens. I want to stay here, talk to you, and get to know you."

Their meeting was why she came, why she spent so much time getting ready, and why she stood in front of him so he could see how exceptional she was. She looked at him, and now he saw vulnerable with a slight touch of fear in her eyes. He wanted to say more. He knew they were both wounded. They were coming off relationships they ended, but the pain was still there, even if the wounds were self-inflicted. You cannot spend that much time with someone on the most intimate of terms and walk away unscathed. To heal their wounds, they had to take a chance. He was willing, but was she?

She continued to study him closely for a moment, then smiled. "So, you were a frat rat with Henry in college." She was willing. She was ready to engage in the timeless game men and women play.

Dave pretended to look hurt, "I was in a fraternity, but I'm not a frat rat." then he continued, "I know exactly what Henry told you about me. He said I was a naïve idealist."

She added, "He also said you are one of the few people he trusts and his best friend. He thinks quite a lot of you."

"Are you impressed?" He smiled his most charming boyish smile.

She laughed again. Her laughter had an enchanting quality that made him want to hear more of it. "What did he tell you about me?"

"He told me you were beautiful, but not that you had such lovely eyes." He could not resist complimenting her eyes any longer.

"Henry told me about that too, the smooth Southern charm. Dial it down. He said you like to read, you're into music, you like to travel, and you backpacked around Europe one summer when you were in med school. I became a flight attendant because I like to travel, I love music, and I spend a lot of time reading."

Without being aware of it, he slid into his pedantic, professorial persona that some of his friends found annoying. "My whole philosophy of life has been shaped by the books I've read. For example, I learned that good must confront evil, but both are often consumed in the process: like the joining of matter and antimatter." He considered himself a student of the nature of man as well as a student of medicine.

"Tolkien. Who else influenced you?" She became interested in what he had to say.

"Dickens taught me ignorance and want are the underlying causes of most of the suffering in a society." Dave's focus shifted from her beauty to what she thought about the issues he considered important. Henry told him there was more to her than her looks, and he wanted to find out who she really was.

"What writers influenced you the most?" Her whole demeanor changed: she was engaged with him now, but like his friends, she found the way he lectured instead of having a conversation annoying.

"Michener, Melville, Steinbeck, Colleen McCullough, Thomas Cahill, Hemingway...."

She interrupted him. "Hemingway! He was a misogynistic chauvinist who glorified war." Her eyes flashed and he realized they could be weaponized.

He countered with, "A Farewell to Arms and For Whom the Bell Tolls are both antiwar. The thing about the Hemingway hero is that although he is damaged, he continues the struggle even in the face of impossible odds."

"That's such a male thing, an excuse you men use to justify your macho actions. Hemingway was a narcissist who didn't portray women well in his books or treat them well in his personal life. The same goes for Dickens, he didn't handle women well in his life or his writing."

"I don't have a problem handling women correctly, and I definitely treat them well." He smiled mischievously.

She interrupted him. "Knock it off. If you can't get your dick out of the way long enough to have a conversation with a woman, then I guess you are a Hemingway man." She started to walk away.

He had mis-stepped badly. He went after her. "I'm sorry, but you're so beautiful...."

She turned back to face him. "You mean if a woman is attractive, she's probably not educated enough or well-read enough to have a discussion with you?"

He mis-stepped again, but he was who he was, and he was not going to become a fabrication of himself to seduce her. He wanted more than that from her. He wanted an honest connection. "Look, I'll put my male part away. See, it's gone, I'm totally dickless. Please, let's stay here and continue to talk." He pleaded.

Her eyes softened as she looked at him. "I'm sorry, but don't disappoint me by being another player looking to hook up. After what Henry told me, I expected more than that from you." She smiled. "And I doubt seriously that you're dickless." Then she continued in a matter-of-fact tone, "But you should know, I'm interested in what's above your shoulders, not what's below your waist."

Her smile faded and she moved close to him. "Are we trying too hard? All that discussion seemed stilted." He sensed a sadness about her and realized it had been there all along lurking beneath the surface. She didn't hide her vulnerability but exposed her feelings to him. "I broke up with a guy a few months ago, and Henry told me you left a girl behind when you moved here. Is that why he introduced us? Did he push us together because he felt sorry for us?" She leaned into him, and the warmth of his body enveloped her as he put his arm around her.

"That's not like Henry, but even if you are right, I want to give us a chance." Her face was turned to his, and her eyes were inviting now. She let down her protective barriers and opened up to him. The dining room was full of people who knew her but not him; yet it was obvious to everyone she was not interested in greetings, nor was he interested in introductions. They stood there quietly for a moment, then continued to talk. They were both bright and inquisitive; they had read the same books, they had developed the same core values, and they shared the same view of the world. They enjoyed agreeing on, or disagreeing on, and debating a wide variety of subjects as their budding connection grew into a full flower. Their warm beers sat abandoned on the table as that flower formulated into the intangible chemistry that develops between a man and a woman. They were near the inflection point of their percolating chemistry, when a man walked up behind her, wrapped his arms around her, and whispered in her ear. "Hello, Gorgeous." She tried to pull away while looking back to see who it was, then she relaxed, and put her hands on his arms as he held her. "Phillip!" Dave was instantly jealous.

Phillip was in his early thirties, handsome, slender, and well dressed. *Henry said there were a lot of men after her, and this guy is not only one of them, he's already been with her. He has his hands all over her, and it's obvious by the way she's responding, she's been in his arms before.* Dave was crushed and his aspirations along with the anticipation that had been building in him poured out to pool in a puddle at her feet. He stood in front of them mute; looking and feeling extremely foolish like an amateur who was supplanted by a professional.

There was another man with Phillip; older, shorter, and heavy set. "Phil and Bob, this is Doctor David Cameron. He and Henry were roommates in college, and he recently moved here to do his internship at University Hospital. Dave, this is Phil and Bob. They're a married couple who live next door and they own one of the most exclusive clothing stores in the city."

Couple! Married! He's gay! Jesus Christ! I'm insanely jealous over a woman I just met and a gay guy. How did I get hooked so deep, so quick? He looked at her standing in front of him laughing in Phil's arms and knew. *It's her, it's everything about her. I've lost myself to her, and the hook is set very deep indeed.*

"Excuse us from barging in like this since it's obvious you two are in heat." Phil kept his arms around her.

"I know you think you're being funny Phil, but I just met Dave, and I don't want him to get the wrong impression of me." She freed herself from Phil and moved back toward Dave.

"I could never get the wrong impression of you. I think you're perfect." He blurted out in his consternation without thinking.

"See Gorgeous, he would never mistake our fun for anything other than that; just fun, right Dave?" Phil looked at him, not at her. "Looks, brains, and manly build; just look at those shoulders! God, he's Dudley Do Right. I wouldn't be surprised if his front tooth sparkles when he smiles. You deserve someone like him after that skinny, controlling, cold asshole Bar. I've never seen you as happy as you are tonight. Don't be afraid to embrace that happiness."

"You guys are obviously Sharon's friends, so I hope we can be friends, too." Dave stuck his hand out.

Phil took his hand and looked at Sharon, "See, I told you, Dudley Do Right. I'm sure he wants to embrace your happiness. Let him. See what it's like to be with someone decent instead of a narcissistic sociopath."

"Bob and Phil don't like Bar because he's just a tad homophobic." She laughed and leaned into Dave so he could put his arm around her waist again.

"It's not that. We deal with that all the time. It's the way he treated you." Phil turned his attention back to Dave. "He treated her like she was nothing more than a hood ornament, and only there for show. He is the great Bar; smarter than you, superior to you in every way, and look at the gorgeous woman he's with."

Bob added, "You two have been talking for some time, Dave. What were you talking about?"

"We were talking about literature, art, and travel." Dave was not sure where this conversation was going, and he wanted to get back to Sharon.

But Bob persisted. "You're an educated man, Dave. Did she hold her own with you on those topics?"

"Of course." He looked at Sharon and smiled.

"Bar controlled everything she did and said. He never let her express an opinion and if she did, he belittled and humiliated her. He only wanted to display her assets to enhance his image. She was there to edify him and prove what a man he was, nothing more." Bob was getting worked up.

Dave could not control his jealousy. "Why did you stay with him?"

"They tend to be a little dramatic. It wasn't that bad. Bar looks like Ichabod Crane, and he gets off more on tormenting people than … ah

16

… anything else. He'd rather do things to other people to see how they react … than ah …." She didn't finish and looked down sheepishly.

Dave felt a surge of emotion for her and took her in his arms. She looked up at him as he held her. "Now, the last thing I want to talk about or think about tonight is Bar. He is gone and forgotten, and I don't want to hear any more about him." He pulled her to him. Their bodies fit together perfectly, and the feel of her body against his sent a rush deep into his core.

"Don't paint me as drama queens, Sharon. You know we're telling the truth." Phil looked at them and realized they were not aware of anyone else as they held each other. "Do you two want to stay here and continue to entertain the dining room with your foreplay, or would you like to give it a rest for a while, and join us for a couple of bottles of good Champagne."

Sharon was a little flushed as she freed herself from Dave, turned and hit Phil lightly in the chest with her fist. "That's enough." She looked back at Dave.

"Sure." He nodded.

"Let us adjourn to the back room." Phil and Bob walked away together.

Dave started to follow them, but she held him back. "Wait, how do you really feel about gay men?"

"I thought it was obvious." Dave turned to her.

"You're very smooth. That could have been an act for my benefit. Those two guys have always been there for me. There's not a mean or devious bone in their bodies; they're kind, generous, and caring. Straight guys can be very conflicted about gay men." Her eyes were flat, and he sensed further explanation was required.

"I believe in freedom. I believe if you don't harm anyone else, you should be free to do what you want. People have been doing what they do since before we climbed down from the trees. Love is love as far as I'm concerned."

She stepped up to him, put her hands on his shoulders, let them slide slowly down to his upper arms, pulled herself against him, and kissed him. When the kiss was over, she looked directly into his eyes, and he could feel the warmth turn to heat.

They caught up with Phil and Bob at a room on the right side of the hall. "What took you so long?"

"We're slow walkers." Sharon took Dave's arm.

"I thought you might be administering a gay tolerance test to Dave." Phil looked intently at Dave.

"That too." She smiled.

"Did he pass?" Bob asked.

"He is an A student." She squeezed his arm.

Dave looked at Sharon. "There's only one problem, I have impure thoughts about my teacher."

"I don't blame you. I have impure thoughts about her, and I am gay. I can only imagine how she must affect a straight guy." Phil opened the door to a dimly lit room with a surround sound system and a wide screen TV on a shelf complex near the door, but no furniture. Instead, the floor was covered with cushions and pillows.

Bob had two bottles of Champagne. "I hate to drink good Champagne from plastic, but...." He popped the cork on one of the bottles and poured each of them a glass. They clinked plastic glasses and relaxed in the cushions to listen to the music. Bob was very attentive; constantly refilling Sharon's and Dave's glasses until the Champagne was finished. When their glasses were finally empty, they fell back in the cushions and did not move for some time as the music washed over them.

Fleetwood Mac's Sentimental Lady reached out of the component sound system and touched them as they lay in the cushions floating on the Champagne. He moved over her, kissed her, and lingered, as his hands roamed over her body. He rolled onto his back, pulled her with him without breaking the kiss, and continued to caress her body as she slid her arms around his neck.

Phil was watching them. "You two need to get a room"

"My room is next door." She untangled herself from him.

"Are you sure?" He asked.

She stood up and adjusted her skirt. "I'm sure. Wait until you try to stand up."

"I'm having trouble just sitting up. Some gay guy gave me a hell of a lot of Champagne." Dave struggled to his feet.

"Goodnight, guys." Sharon said as she walked toward the door.

Phil reached out to Dave. "Hold on, I think you're a good guy, Dave, but you need to understand she's not someone you can simply use and discard. She's been hurt enough. She needs to be cherished by someone who values her." Dave nodded to Phil and joined Sharon in the hall. His heart was pounding because he was about to have sex with the woman of his dreams, his fantasy woman, and she was real, standing right in front of him soft, warm, and willing.

As they passed the opening to the living room, Henry was still sitting on the couch with Sherry, but Mike had joined them. Henry started to say something as they passed but realized there was nothing to say. Mike's eyes never left Sharon as he stood up and followed them out. He watched them walk to the other house from the front porch, came back in, and went straight to the keg.

Sherry watched them leave, too. She liked Sharon, even though she was a little jealous of her, but Sharon wasn't her concern. Henry was. She had plans for her future, and he was at the center of those plans. They would marry and move to New York City where he would become a well-known internist. With their money and connections, she could become a New York socialite, and join the most exclusive, elite social circle in the country. This Dave person could not interfere with that. Henry seemed different since he arrived. It was this Dave person she needed to be concerned about.

Sharon's room reflected her personality; it was simple, classy and tasteful. He waited by the bed as the hauntingly romantic sound of a solo saxophone drifted through the room, and she walked back to stand in front of him. She removed her top slowly one button at a time, unzipped her skirt, let it fall to the floor, stepped out of it gracefully, then used her thumbs to remove her thong. "I don't want you to be disappointed, so you should know I am not very experienced at this." Her eyes were wide and bright as she stood in front of him.

He could not stop looking at her incredible body as he fumbled trying to pull his T-shirt over his head and stumbled trying to slide his jeans off. She felt tense and there was a slight trembling in her body when he held her in his arms. He pulled back from her "We don't have to do this if you're not ready. We can wait." She responded to what he said by pressing her body against his. That was all the encouragement he needed.

A woman's body is like a musical instrument that can be played to produce cords of ecstasy. Dave learned to play the female body from some very hedonistic, pleasure-seeking women focused only on their own gratification, and they taught him how to play it properly. Sharon's body was exquisite, and he used all his skills to play it with the care an exquisite instrument deserves, making sure the chords he struck produced notes of intense pleasure for her. Good sex is like good jazz. Each player takes a part until they come together in blended harmonic perfection.

He nibbled her ear lobe and kissed her neck before continuing down, brushing her skin lightly with his lips. Her breathing became rapid and shallow as he took her to a place she had never been before. She threw her arms out, digging her fingers into the bedding as her chest blushed a vivid salmon color, then she bucked wildly, and cried out as the salmon flush turned to deep red blotches. Finally, she collapsed on the bed completely limp. She lay very still with her eyes closed and she was barely breathing. Her hair was spread out around her calm expressionless face and her whole body was totally relaxed. She reminded him of the rendition of an enchanted goddess he had once seen on the cover of a book.

She opened her eyes, pulled him down, and kissed him; a deep, lustful kiss that continued until she pushed him over. What she lacked in experience; she compensated for with enthusiasm. He rolled her onto her back, she wrapped her arms and legs around him, and they kissed again, another lustful passionate kiss that continued as they moved together. "Keep your eyes open." He whispered.

Looking into her enchanting eyes, it felt as if he was falling into her through her eyes. If the eyes are the windows to the soul, her windows were wide open and welcoming. She clutched him tighter with her arms and legs as both their bodies convulsed violently. He started to move, but she hugged him back to her, and they lay joined together until she spoke. "I've never experienced anything like that before. I never dreamed it could be that wonderful."

He moved onto his back, and she leaned up on her elbow with her hand on the side of her head and looked at him. "I know I acted like one tonight, but I'm not a slut. I've never done anything like this before. I don't screw every man I meet. I don't even have sex with the men I date. You may not believe that because of the way I acted tonight, but it's true

She sat up. "Henry called me and told me he wanted me to meet his college roommate tonight at the party. I told him I wasn't going to the party. He told me I had to go and meet you. He built you up so much, I decided to go, and see if anyone could be that great." She laid back down. "I put what I have on display to see if you could get past my looks and connect with who I am. Most men don't even try. I wanted to test you." She added in a small, soft voice. "Obviously, you passed the test."

She sat up again. "You look dangerous with your vivid blue eyes and long blond hair, and you frightened me a little at first. But what made me give you a chance was your confidence, not arrogance or cockiness, but understated confidence." She continued. "You didn't talk about sports, your car, or yourself, the way most Southern men do. You actually sought out who I was, and you seemed to be exactly who Henry said you were. Of course, it was Phil who pushed me over the edge by telling me to let go and indulge myself with a man like you: that and all the Champagne. So, I let go and he was right, something wonderful happened, but I don't want you to think I act like this with every man I meet."

She was so open and vulnerable, he sat up and took her in his arms. "How foolish are you? We're in the afterglow of the best sex I've ever had. I've never experienced anything like that, either. We had an amazing experience that's all that matters."

"Really?" She looked at him in disbelief, reached out, touched his lips with her fingertips, traced them all the way around, then looked down again. "I suppose you want to go now."

"Do you want me to go?"

"No, but if you want to go, I'll understand." She said in a guarded voice, then she added in a soft low voice, "Bar never stayed with me after we had sex. He always went back to his room and left me feeling alone and used. I've never felt protected and secure with a man, like I feel with you, I want to stay."

He held her close, kissed her, cradled her in his arms, and they settled into the bed together. Dave was high on Champagne, but he was even higher on the whole night, so he lay awake for a while holding her soft warm body against his, listening to her quiet breathing.

His high school friends had finished college, married, and bought homes, while at twenty-six, he was still basically in school, and living in apartments. In college, he spent his afternoons in labs while his fraternity brothers were enjoying all college had to offer. But that was nothing compared to the two basic science years of medical school. Then came his clerkship along with more stress, sleeplessness, and fatigue. When he took Medicine, he was up at six, at the hospital by seven, and he stayed there all night when his team was on call. He was grilled about his patients by his attendings, attended classes, and took tests. It had taken discipline and a single-minded adherence to purpose for him to reach this point in his life.

Monday he would begin the next phase of his training and he had no allusions. He knew it would be worse than anything he had been through so far, but tonight, as he held Sharon in his arms, none of that mattered, because he was literally sleeping with the woman of his dreams.

He woke up in an excited state, but she was still asleep. He tried to think about something else, but that was impossible with her in bed next to him. In homo saps, as his college biology professor used to say, and not without good cause, the female has secondary sex characteristics that indicate fertility. Those characteristics attract the visual male who wants to spread his genes with a fertile female. Her secondary sex characteristics were right up against him, and he was ready to spread his genes.

She woke up with a start because a man was in her bed, but as the sleep began to clear from her mind, she remembered last night, and a warm wave of contentment swept over her. The feeling was new to her, but she liked it. She liked the way he made her feel last night, and she liked the way she felt now. She continued to be sexually free with him because she wanted more of both feelings. "Someone must have had a good dream." She pulled him to her, and they had sweet morning sex, and although it was nothing like the night before, in its own way, it was just as satisfying.

She whispered in his ear, "I am starving. I didn't eat before the party. Let's go make breakfast." She put on a short, sheer robe, he put on his jeans, and they padded downstairs barefoot. "I can make bacon and eggs. You start the coffee, set the table, get some orange juice, and make toast." He came up behind her while she was cooking the eggs, caressed her breasts, nuzzled her neck, and slid his hand down until she rotated in his arms. "Stop that or I will get distracted and burn the eggs. Behave yourself or you won't get any breakfast." She wiggled out of his arms and turned back to the eggs, but her breathing had changed, and she felt a tingling from his touch. "Last night I realized I have been missing something. You may be exactly what I need. A man who knows how to handle a woman and treat her well." She smiled, then laughed out loud.

When the eggs were finished, they sat down to eat, and she decided to find out more about him. "I've never … been with a man … who made me … feel … I've never been with anyone like you." She blushed and looked down, wondering who he really was. "Are you a gentle idealist, like Henry said, or is there something more about you? I know you played football and that's a violent game. Do you have a violent side? Are you who you appear to be, or do you wear a mask like most men do; a mask that hides a part of you?"

"Did Henry tell you I played football?" He looked worried.

"You didn't get those shoulders, arms, and that tight rear from playing golf." Her response was matter of fact.

"Does it make a difference that I did?" He asked in a quiet voice.

"Not if you're over it, not the football, obviously you don't play football anymore, but the violence I mean. Are you over the violence? And please tell me you don't hunt and kill beautiful woodland creatures."

"I liked playing football, but I'm not a violent person. I liked the 'game' part of it, the competition, and the attention, you know, the 'give me the ball, and watch me go' part of it." He paused. "But I quit playing to concentrate on school. I don't hunt, and I don't wear a mask. I don't hide who I am. I value my integrity too much. There's nothing phony about me. I'm comfortable with who I am."

She got up and picked up the plates. "It's getting late, and I have to fly tomorrow, I need to wash my hair and do some things."

"Can I see you tonight?"

"Yes, but I have to get to bed early. I have a morning flight." She looked directly into his eyes, arousing him in ways he had never felt before.

"I have no problem with us getting to bed early." He reached for her, but she shied away. "Don't worry. I'll go. Not willingly, but I'll go."

They exchanged phone numbers, he gave her his address, and she told him she would pick up some takeout for dinner on the way to his apartment. He kissed her goodbye and walked back to the other house. A nice-looking, thin aesthetic looking young man in glasses was in the dining room cleaning up from the party. "Hi, I am Dave Cameron. Is Henry here?"

"I know who you are. I'm Harvin, one of Henry's roommates. You know you crushed a lot of guys' hopes last night. I was extremely impressed. You just walked in and walked out with her. You really let the air out of their balloons." Dave ignored what he said, so he continued, "Henry went to Sherry's last night after the party, but your friend's upstairs. He moved in this morning. He's a little hung over. It turned into a hell of a party after you left, but I guess you're not sorry you missed it. Let's go up and I'll show you Mike's room."

Mike was sprawled on his bed. "So, how was last night and did you have breakfast this morning too?"

"She's amazing. I've never been with anyone like her." Dave had a faraway look in his eyes. "I'm not even sure she's real. She's like a fantasy I conjured up from my dreams or some ethereal being from another world."

"I saw her. She's really hot, and I take it she's as tasty as she looks." Mike wasn't going to let it go.

Dave came back to reality. "And she's smart, sophisticated, classy: the whole package."

"So, she's not a slut, she just dresses like one and acts like one. If she isn't a slut, she sure was wearing a slut's uniform last night. Do you actually think it was your boyish good looks and irresistible charm that caused her to lose her head then start giving you head that quick?" Mike's voice dripped with venom.

"Knock it off." Dave tried to change the subject. "I came by to talk to Henry and see if you were moving in here. Henry isn't here, and you're moved in, so I'm going to take off. I need to read the stuff we got at orientation and fill out all the forms. Have you done that yet?"

"I spent yesterday getting it done. I get it. You like this slut. But don't kid yourself, you're far from the first one down that road. I'll bet there are ruts in it up to your knees. That field has been plowed many times before you plowed it. You want to get a beer later?"

"No, I'm seeing her again tonight. I want to spend as much time with her as possible before we're tied up at the hospital." Dave changed the subject again. "Are you worried about being responsible for your patients instead of just watching someone else make the decisions?"

"No, we're ready. We'll be fine. See you later." Mike dismissed him.

Dave did not understand that Mike was more envious of him than he could have possibly imagined. Mike spent a significant amount of his emotional energy on envy. He had a higher class ranking than Dave, he matched with a straight Medicine internship at University Hospital, while Dave had to apply for a rotating position. He excelled at everything he attempted, yet it was Dave who hardly ever slept alone when they lived together, and it was Dave who spent last night with the most desirable woman he had ever seen; including the airbrushed, photoshopped models on the fantasy sex website he frequented.

His new roommates further augmented his discontent. Harvin and Henry were both trust fund babies who attended prep school together, and were members of the elite wealthy class he so wanted to be a part of. Even George, who seemed average in every way, was from an upper-class background. All of them were with very attractive women last night, and even though there were unattached women at the party; he ended up alone, he went home alone, and he slept alone; but not Dave; no, Dave seemed to always have a bed partner.

Dave left Mike to seethe in his jealousy, drove to his apartment, and called Henry. "Hi Dave, what's up?"

"I don't know what to say. Last night was the most magical night of my life."

"Really?" Henry replied dryly.

"Have you been talking to Mike?"

"No, Mike has been talking to me, and anyone else willing to listen."

"I got some of that this morning."

"I don't think you do get it, Dave. He trash-talked Sharon, the woman you were with, and you for being with her. I don't want anything to do with him, and you should avoid him too."

"I know he's a bit resentful of those of us he sees as more fortunate, but he has a good heart." Dave was loyal to his friends, so he defended Mike.

"All I am saying is watch your back with him, Dave. He will stab you in it the first chance he gets. There are people in this world who are toxic. When you identify one, you need to get as far from them as possible, as fast as possible. That's what you need to do with Mike because he's toxic."

"I didn't call to talk about Mike. I called to talk about Sharon. How did you know we would connect like that?" Dave changed the subject because he knew Henry was probably right.

"I knew you would like each other because you look into the pool of the other person and see your own reflection. You read the same books, you are both attractive, well Sharon is drop-dead gorgeous, you both like music and art, you both like to travel, I could go on. I thought you two would connect because you would be connecting with yourselves." He laughed. "I have to admit, I didn't know you would literally connect physically quickly."

"So, it wasn't magic but psychology. I don't believe it. I believe it was pure magic. You know, Henry, sometimes it is best not to see the wires and believe in the magic." Dave believed some things happened for reasons that were outside the realm of physical nature.

"There's no magic. There are always wires, even if you don't see them. Science is behind everything. You know that. You are a biologist. It's all science and math." Henry scoffed.

"I'll bet you enjoy telling kids there's no Easter Bunny. I want to talk about Sharon, and you make me talk about Mike. I want to thank you for a magical night, and you tell me it's all psychology." Dave believed last night was one of those things that had no explanation.

"You are a biologist, Dave. Do I really need to explain to you why you're attracted to her? She's an evolved modern woman. You have brains and brawn, the perfect combination for someone like her. Your biology and your dynamics made the connection, not magic. It was simply the perfect biological and psychological pairing."

"It was also fueled by a lot of Champagne. I think the alcohol took her inhibitions to the floor." Dave was too happy to let Henry bring him back to reality.

"Only a person as highly intelligent and intuitive as I am could have orchestrated such a perfect pairing." But Henry wondered about last night. Sharon was usually so reserved and sophisticated, but the way she was dressed, then jumping right into bed with Dave? It was uncharacteristic of her, and he couldn't help questioning his own hypothesis. Could there be something in the equation he wasn't aware of?

"I get it, but I still want to thank you for the most wonderful night of my life, regardless of the biology, psychology, or whatever behind it. I'll see you on Monday."

Dave spent the rest of the afternoon filling out the forms from orientation. Later he set two places in front of the stools at the counter between the kitchen and front room: he didn't have a table and chairs. He remade the bed with clean sheets, put fresh towels in the bathroom, and scented candles in the rooms. He drove to the supermarket to buy a bottle of decent white wine, a six-pack of beer, and some flowers; then he wrapped the flowers in tissue paper and put them on one of the oversized bean bags. When he was satisfied everything was perfect, he took a shower, shaved, used a lot of cologne, and dressed.

He sat down in the other bean bag and looked around his apartment with a sense of satisfaction. Along with his medical books, there was a component surround sound system, and a flat screen TV on a large shelf complex beside the door. Two big bean bags were on the opposite wall with a small wicker table between them. There were sliding glass doors that led to a balcony with a view of the pool area. The bathroom was past the kitchen on the left and the bedroom was behind the front room on the right.

His medical school had an agreement with a private hospital to hire medical students during the summer to cover their staff's vacations. He worked as a urology tech his first summer. After he had pharmacology in his sophomore year, he worked as a medication nurse on a med-surg floor. The summer after he had medicine his junior year, he worked as a CCU nurse. He spent some of the money he made on travel, bought things he wanted, like the television and sound system, and saved the rest. When he graduated from med school in mid-May, he did not have to report for his internship until late June, so he worked as a charge nurse in the ED on the eleven-to-seven shift. Six weeks of ER charge nurse's salary gave him enough money for the move, the apartment, and to trade his car in on a new sports car.

While he was waiting, he thought about what Henry said. He understood he was a complex biochemical, electrophysiologic organism, and even the thoughts he was currently having were the results of neurotransmitters stimulation and depolarizing cells in his brain. He also knew emotions were probably stored in those cells in some way, but he felt something beyond that transpired last night.

The doorbell rang. She was standing at the door, her hip cocked to one side with her elbow resting on it, her arm extended palm up, holding a bag with Chinese letters on it. She smiled and said, "I come bearing Chinese takeout." He had forgotten how striking she was and seeing her completely unnerved him. She was dressed in a light green cropped T-shirt, dark green shorts, and white strappy wedge sandals that made her shapely legs look as if they went on forever.

"Well, are you going to invite me in? If not, there were a couple of cute guys checking me out in the parking lot, and I bet one of them will invite me in if you don't." He looked down the stairs to see two men walk by looking up. She walked past him to the kitchen, put the food bag's contents in the oven, set it to warm, and saw the flowers. "Dave! Do you have a vase? We need to put them in water." He put the flowers in a water pitcher, placed it on the counter between the place settings, poured her a glass of wine, and got himself a beer. "Are you going to light the candles?" She settled into the bean bags where the flowers had been.

Finally, he spoke, "I was, but you smell too good. What are you wearing?" He sat down in the other bean bag.

"Chanel." She looked at him under her eyebrows as she took a sip of wine. Soft music was playing low in the background so they could talk, but they both knew why she was there, they both knew what they wanted, and they both knew it had nothing to do with talking. They went to the kitchen and filled their plates with vegetable fried rice, Peking duck, and egg rolls. When they finished eating, they got more wine and beer, went back to the bean bags, he changed the music, turned the volume up, and music filled the apartment.

"I want to dance." She stood up and danced to the middle of the room. Dave was a good dancer, but he recognized at once that she was a trained dancer and stopped. "You're a dancer."

"Twelve years of ballet from the first grade through my senior year in high school." She curved her arms in front of her and did a tight spin, turning her head to spot as she spun. "Now, put your hands lightly on my waist." She lifted her arms above her head, stood on one foot, used the other to kick-turn in his hands, stopped facing him, put her arms around his neck, and threw her head back laughing. "We just did a pas de deux."

She was a dancer. That explained everything. Her gracefulness, how lithe she was, her perfect legs, her amazing body, the way she moved, her confidence, how she presented herself, her style, everything. It was all clear to him now.

"I haven't danced since college, and I haven't done ballet since high school. Who are you, Dave Cameron? How do you have such an effect on me? What's your sign? Where did you come from? How did you make it? Why do I see myself so differently when I am with you, and why do I feel free to do whatever I want?" Dave thought about his conversation with Henry, but he refused to see any wires. It was magic, pure magic, he was sure of it.

"Why did you stop dancing?" He slid his arms around her.

"Dance is an expression of joy. Something happened that took the joy out of my life." A dark shadow clouded her features and he saw sadness in her again. "Besides, I was too tall, and I knew I wasn't going to make a career out of it, but I don't want to talk about that now." She laughed, "In fact, I don't want to talk at all." She put her arms around his neck, jumped up, and locked her legs around his waist.

It was a repeat of the night before, but now there was no awkwardness or uncertainty. They took their time and enjoyed every aspect of their pas de deux. They were a tight sexual duet now, playing each other, and playing off each other to produce harmonic ecstasy. She screamed because he did not stop but pushed her until she convulsed so hard it seemed as if she was having a seizure. For Dave, it was so intense it was almost painful, and he cried out as he clung to her. Afterwards, they lay silently in bed with his arms around her and her head on his chest. At last, she said, "What time is it?"

"It's nine. It's finally dark outside. I can't imagine being in this bed without you tonight." He pulled her closer.

"I need to go. I have to get up at four, if I get to bed by ten, I'll only get six hours of sleep, and I have a hard trip tomorrow." She got up, went to the bathroom, and when she came back, she was dressed.

He pulled on his jeans, followed her to the front room, and held her, reluctant to let her go. "Can I see you when you get back?"

She whispered, "Please, I have to go now," and she pushed herself out of his arms. "I'll call you when I get back." He followed her to her car, gave her the flowers and kissed her, then cautioned her several times to drive safely before she drove away. He missed her by the time her taillights disappeared.

Back in his apartment, the room seemed empty and lifeless without her glow and vitality. He had only known her for two days, but he was terribly lonely without her. When he went to bed, he could smell her in the bedding, Chanel. He drifted off to sleep with her fragrance producing images in his head.

When he woke Monday morning and his mind cleared, he smelled her on the sheets. *I'm not going to wash my sheets. I want my bed to smell like her.* He showered, got dressed and drove to the Hospital.

His phone rang late that night.

"Hi, Dave," she said in a low husky voice that made him ache for her. "How was your trip?"

"It sucked. The first leg to LA was fine but LAX was so backed up we were held for hours. LAX's backup caused the whole West Coast to hold flights and that made our flight even later. I just walked in, and I am dead tired."

"Can we spend the weekend of the Fourth together?" There was a touch of pleading in his voice.

"Really? Are you asking me for a date?" She said in the same low husky voice again.

"Yes, I guess. We just met … I mean. I don't know." Her voice unsettled him.

She dropped her voice another octave. "We know each other about as intimately as two people can know each other, and you're asking me to spend the weekend with you. Don't you think we're a bit past the 'asking for a date' stage?"

"I know … I know how I feel … I wasn't sure how you … how you felt." He was flustered and stumbled over his words.

"Really, after last night you don't know how I feel? You must not be as smart as I thought you were." She teased him.

Dave was as happy as a teenage boy with his first girlfriend. "Sherry is going to organize a picnic for the concert and fireworks, then we're going to have a party at the park house afterwards. Your roommates and their dates are invited too. Can we spend the night at my apartment when you get back tomorrow? It's my last night before I start."

"What time should I come over? I get back at five and I'm fine for the weekend. I don't have another long trip or a layover for a week."

"I hate layovers. I hate whoever invented layovers, and I hate the airline for having layovers." He responded a bit harshly.

She laughed at him. "I'll get you a copy of my schedule."

"It's not that, it's the layover thing. I'll bet you get hit on by every pilot, copilot, and first officer you fly with, not to mention the passengers. You couldn't walk from your car to my apartment last night without some guys following you. It's someone laying over you on a layover that's bothering me." He was not happy about the layover thing.

"Are you jealous?" She sounded surprised.

"No, I am not jealous. If I were jealous, I would be an insecure, pathetic loser. No one wants to be with an insecure, pathetic loser." He tried, without success, to cover up his emotions.

"You're jealous." She sounded amused.

"OK, I am jealous, and I hate myself. See what you have done to me, you've turned me into a green monster. The thought of you with some pilot, first office, or passenger on a layover is killing me. I won't be able to sleep with you on a layover. I will be up all night wondering who is laying over you." Dave was not amused.

"I'm happy being with you, Dave, and only with you. I don't sleep around. If that changes, I'll tell you. All I ask is the same commitment from you. I expect you to protect me by not sleeping with someone else while we're together. Is that clear enough for you? We're in a kind of fantasy bubble now: let's make the most of it. Let's just be happy and enjoy the moment. I'm committed to telling you if I date someone else, or sleep with someone else, and that's all the commitment I want from you. I'm coming off an obsessive, controlling relationship, and I am not going down that road again. Also, regardless of what you say, I sense a violent side to you, and I certainly don't want to deal with that." She said "again", under her breath.

"Does that mean we are going steady? Do you want my medical school ring to wear around your neck on a gold chain?" He quipped.

Now, she was not amused. "I don't know why I like you. I tell you how I feel, and you make a joke out of it." Then she used her low husky voice again. "No one else is going to lay over me, Dave. I only want you to lay over me. I'll let you know if that changes." They said goodnight, he put some music on, and tried to settle down, but she had a powerful hold on him, and that hold went deeper than the sex.

Before going to bed, he turned on the classic movie station and watched Twelve O'clock High, an old black and white movie about the bomber raids over Germany during the Second World War. The movie was disturbing because it demonstrated that no matter how strong someone was, they could be broken by stress and responsibility. That caused his thoughts to shift to the coming year. Would he be able to manage being the doctor in charge, or would he be broken like the Gregory Peck character in the movie? He did not sleep well that night and woke up early.

Dave and Henry met the two outgoing interns and the four of them went to breakfast. He learned from one of the interns, "Your attending is Doctor Finkel, the head of the Department of Endocrinology, and he hates interns. He believes the internship year should be eliminated and residency should start right after graduation. He wants one year of basic sciences pushed down to college level and those courses made prerequisites for entrance into medical school. That would free up the last year of medical school to become the internship year. You would do your internship in your senior year of medical school then start your residency right after graduation. His plan would add an extra year to our clinical training." The other intern added, "If he's anything, it's not fair, but don't worry, Dave. Sheffield writes the recommendations for rotators. All you two have to do is kiss Finkel's ass and worship his

magnificence." After breakfast they reviewed all their charts, familiar-
ized themselves with the treatment plans, then introduced themselves
to the patients.

Dave completed his day and drove home to wait for Sharon. He
heard her at the door, opened it, and she was standing there holding
her travel case and hanging bag. He pulled her in, took her travel case
and hanging bag, dropped them on the floor, and kissed her. "All I could
think about all day was you, and I couldn't wait to see you." He kissed
her and held her close until he carried her into the bedroom and laid
her down on the bed. "It's fantasy bubble time." He kissed her again,
then pulled her top over her head and threw it aside. "Dave!" He found
the zipper for her shorts, unzipped them, and pulled them off, "Dave!"
He stripped off his T-shirt and jeans. In no time she was crying out
and using a few profane words in connection with Dave's name. "Did
that meet your fantasy bubble expectations?"

"Pretty much." She laughed dryly. "Are we going to eat something
tonight?"

He sat back and watched her. "There is a little family-run Mexican
place only a few blocks from here."

She sensed his thoughts as he watched her dress. "Don't objectify
me. I objectify myself enough. I know how I look, and I admit I use
my looks, but I put too much of my self-worth in my looks. I depend
on them too much. I know it sounds counter intuitive, but my looks
get in my way. Men don't take me seriously. They only want to screw
me. Women are jealous of me and hate me, so they are condescending
to me."

He came up behind her and kissed her neck. "But there's so much
more to you than your looks. Your real value is in who you are."

In bed that night, she reflected on who Dave was. Like Henry said,
he was naïve and idealistic. She was idealistic too, but she was much
more mature than he was. He was still such a boy. When she was
younger, she dreamed of having a lover like Shelley or Keats; intelligent,

educated, sensitive, and cultured. Dave was not what she had pictured at all. He was intelligent, educated, sensitive, and cultured, but he was a powerful man with a cut body, broad shoulders, and strong arms who lived by a code she did not completely understand. She never dreamed she would have a lover who could make her cry out in carnal pleasure. She smiled and almost laughed out loud thinking about that. He slept soundly that night because he knew with her in his life, he was ready for the coming year.

Chapter 2

The Medicine Wards

It was dark when he joined the morning commute traffic, but he could see the other driver's shadowy faces in the faint glow of their dashboard lights. *Am I one of them? I'm going to work like they are, but this is the first day of my life as a doctor, does that make me different? I want to be different; I want my life to be different, I want to live an exceptional, well lived life.* The thoughts rushed through his mind like the cars rushing along the expressway beside him.

He hated getting up early, but he liked driving in the early morning hours before dawn. He enjoyed the cool clean feeling of the predawn. It heralded a fresh new day and a new beginning in which anything was possible. Before he reached the hospital, his last thoughts were of Sharon. He pictured her sleeping in his bed with her long hair spread around her lovely face and her perfect form outlined under the sheet.

When he arrived, the campus of University Hospital was brightly lit and brimming with activity in the fading darkness. The automatic doors of the ED silently slid open on the glaring lights, the out-of-tune symphony of sounds, and the sharp smells of the ED. It all hit him in the face with a surge of excitement. He felt a rush of adrenaline as he walked past the triage desk, showed the nurse his ID, and started down the hall for the elevators. He was back in it and the intensity felt good. He took the elevator up to the medicine floor with his heart beating a little faster the way it did before a game, then he walked confidently to the nursing station ready to begin his first day as a doctor.

"We be in it now brother, we be the RD's!" Henry had a big grin on his face. "Were you with Sharon? If you were, I'm surprised you could tear yourself away from her amazing assets and join us here today."

"I was with her, and she's sleeping soundly in my bed while I'm here stomping out disease and saving lives. She and her roommates will be at the party on the Fourth. I tore myself away from her in my warm bed this morning because, like you said, we be the RD's, and we be in it now."

They picked up their lab coats Monday; put their stethoscopes, reflex hammers, dividers, and tuning forks in the pockets and left them in the doctor's station. Now, Dave was more than a little cocky as he donned the mantle of his profession for the first time.

"Are you two ready to stomp out disease and save lives now, or do I need to wait a little longer until you finish working out your social calendar, talking about your girlfriend's assets, and chest bumping each other because you be the RD's, and you be in it now." The nurses in the nurse's station giggled, but the charge nurse standing in door of the doctor's station looked at them without the slightest hint of a smile. She was attractive, young, neat, and starched with her whole being screaming competent and no nonsense.

Dave and Henry looked at each other and answered politely. "Yes, ma'am, we're ready."

A smile appeared because she knew they were not a couple of rowdies like she first thought. "I'm one of the charge nurses on Medicine Three." She established control. "I expect you to address all my nurses with respect, like nurse Jane Pauley here, who pulled up your charts, labs, and reports for you today. In the future you will have to pull up your own charts, labs, and reports. Doctor Tarkington went to school here so he can help you get to know the system, Doctor Cameron. Now Nurse Pauley will answer any questions you have. I need to finish my report."

Nurse Jane Pauley was standing behind the charge nurse. She was older, slightly overweight, friendly, and an intern's ally. "Call me Jane; I like that better than Nurse Pauley, which makes me sound like an old lady. I function as the liaison between the house staff and the nurses, so if you have any problems or questions, come to me first." Dave and Henry grew to like, respect, and depend on Jane. They dubbed her Nurse Jane Fuzzy Wuzzy.

"You each picked up admissions overnight so unless you have any questions, I suggest you get to work." Henry and Dave sat down at their desks to begin their first day as interns. Jane came back with two cups of coffee and a handful of condiments. "Don't expect this again either. Like having your charts pulled up, this is a one-time thing, and my last contribution to your first day."

They reviewed their new patients' charts and made rounds on them before the junior resident walked into the station. He was tall, thin, and pale with a shock of unkempt brown hair and intelligent eyes behind rimless glasses. But it was his crumpled tattersall shirt, knit tie, wrinkled khaki pants, and scuffed brown loafers that caused Dave to look at Henry with raised eyebrows.

"I'm James McDonald, but everyone calls me Jay. I'm the junior resident, and you are Henry and David?"

"I'm Henry."

"I'm Dave, we were college roommates, fraternity brothers, and are best friends so we tend to be a little loose with each other, but we can act like professionals if it is absolutely necessary." Dave smiled as he stuck out his hand.

Jay was saved from further interaction with them by the charge nurse. "Doctor McDonald, I was so glad to hear you were going to be our resident. It is good to see you again. I hope you are doing well."

"It is good to be back, and it is nice to see you again, Carol." Jay fidgeted and shifted his feet as he spoke to her.

"I need to get home and get some sleep. I just wanted to say hello and welcome you back." She smiled at Jay, then walked away briskly.

As soon as she left, the senior resident took her place at the door. "I know Jay, so you two must be Henry and David, I am Ed Walker, the senior resident." His arrival gave Jay an opportunity to regain his composure after his encounter with Nurse Carol. Ed was a nice-looking, well-dressed young man of average height and build, with a smooth, confident manner that made people like him immediately. "It's after seven so I suggest you get started, as my grand pappy used to say, daylight's a burning."

Dave rounded on his patients, then wrote notes and orders on them. His service was typical for a teaching hospital. All of them were admitted because they would not have survived without hospitalization. There was a patient with congestive heart failure due to cardiomyopathy being evaluated for transplant, a liver failure patient with ascites admitted for hospice care, a terminal cancer patient, a patient with stasis dermatitis and chronic cellulitis, plus six others.

The adrenaline and excitement had faded, and Dave was settling into the reality of the situation as he walked to the cafeteria with Henry. "I think we're going to get five to six admits every call and have five to six left."

"I'm going to need roller skates to get through rounds by ten o'clock with that many patients." Henry looked troubled.

"I'm going to do as much as possible the night before. I'm going to go from seven to seven on the days we are not on call, so with call and weekends, that's eighty to a hundred hours a week. I don't think there's any way to do it in less time than that. I can get up at six to be here by seven, and with six hours of sleep, which leaves five hours free on the weeknights we're not on call." Dave had it all figured out.

"Are you scheduling your Medicine rotation around Sharon? Are you two a couple now?" Henry wasn't surprised about them being a couple, but he was surprised by Dave's approach to it.

Dave failed to answer Henry's questions. "Are you going to keep the room at the park house or move in with Sherry?" They went through the line and found a table.

"Sherry has visions of me in a prestigious private practice with her as my wife. I'm not going to marry her or go into private practice, and

I think when she finds that out, she'll break up with me. I'm keeping the room at the park house for when she kicks me out. The bottom line is I need a woman, and I don't have time to find a new one, so I'm keeping my plans to myself, and I'm keeping the room at the park house." Henry looked down at his food and did not look at Dave as he spoke.

Back on the station Dave called Sharon. "Hi, Baby, I can't talk, but can you meet me at my apartment around seven tonight after you get back from your trip."

"I'm leaving for the airport now, but I'll be back in time to meet you at seven." Then she used her husky soft voice, "Since when am I your Baby?"

"Since the minute I first saw you. I have to go now; I'll see you tonight?"

"Do you want coffee, tea, or just me tonight?" She teased in the same voice.

"Just you Baby, and I'll show you how I take my Sharon tonight, but I have to go now. I'll see you at seven, bye."

He heard a female voice from the nurses' station. "How are you going to take your Sharon tonight, Doctor Cameron?"

I need to keep my dick out of the way. He refused to look at Henry.

Dr. Finkel did not arrive until after ten thirty. His personality was so inflated, it penetrated every corner of the room. "I know who you are so we can dispense with introductions. I'm Doctor Aaron Finkel, I'm a full professor of Medicine and head of the Department of Endocrinology." His arrogance was palpable. "I don't want to go over the patients today. You didn't admit them, and you aren't familiar with them yet. Instead, I would like to know what you plan to do with yourself when you finish your training here. Let's start with you, Ed. What are you going to do when you finish your residency?"

Ed wanted to join University Hospital's private medical group and volunteer as a townie to supervise the house staff in the Medicine Clinic.

Finkel liked the part about volunteering to work in the clinic. Dave wondered if Ed threw that in because he knew it would go over well.

"Jay, what about you? What are you going to do when you finish?"

"Academic medicine, I'll look for an entry-level teaching position at a medical school where there is room for advancement." Jay felt comfortable teaching because it was didactic and required a minimum of patient interaction or social discourse.

"Henry, what about you?"

"I am going to apply for a fellowship in Infectious Disease and do research." Another satisfactory answer by Finkel's standards.

He turned to Dave. "And you, David? Why did you apply for a rotating internship and what do you plan to do with it?"

"In order to get a straight medicine internship at a top institution I had to be in the top ten percent of my class and the top ten percent on the National Boards. I wasn't. Doing a rotating internship gives me the opportunity to work my way into a better residency."

Finkel looked intrigued. "And what are you going to do after you finish this better residency?" Finkel leaned toward Dave.

"I want to practice in a rural area where I can be close to nature and take advantage of the outdoors. I want to be the classic small-town doctor. I guess I'm a bit of a throwback."

"A doctor in an urban, university-connected medical group needs different skills from one who practices solo in a rural area. An academic and a researcher need different skills from someone in patient care. This service currently has twenty-four patients, and those twenty-four patients are your priority, but your approach to that priority can vary depending on what you intend to do with your future. Tomorrow, I will meet with you to go over all the patients on this service. I expect your performance to be excellent and I will accept nothing short of excellent."

As they filed out of the station to go to rounds with the chief, Henry turned to Dave. "You gave a good answer on the rotating internship question. He was prepared to climb all over you, but he couldn't argue with what you said. That's why he saved you for last, he was going to grill you, but you shut him down with that answer, at least for now."

They took their places in the front row of the conference room. Sheffield stood at the front of the room rocking back and forth on his feet like a drill instructor about to address his troops. "Are we all here? Good, let's get started. I don't want to discuss the new admissions, instead I want to discuss a case from last year because it illustrates something I want you to learn on your first day. This is the case of a forty-year-old Hispanic woman admitted in extremis with symptoms involving multiple organ systems. A good intern and an excellent resident admitted her. By the time of this conference the working diagnosis was Addison's disease, hypothyroidism, and diabetes. I have one question, and since you two are up," he looked at Dave and Henry in the front row, "what organ participates in all functions of the endocrine system?"

Dave and Henry both answered, "The pituitary."

"Correct, she had panhypopituitarism. She had a million-dollar work up, but the only one who made the correct diagnosis was the student. How did he make the diagnosis: by taking a detailed history? All the doctors took a history, but they failed to ask one question. Why did the student ask the question? Because he was doing a thorough job. They all asked about her pregnancies; she had five pregnancies and five children. The question the student asked that the others failed to ask, was did she have any problems with any of her pregnancies? The answer was yes; she bled heavily with her last delivery, the bleeding couldn't be stopped, and she had to be transfused. So, what happened, team three?"

Dave and Henry shared the answer.

"The blood supply to her pituitary was compromised."

"It was damaged by ischemia."

"Correct. The lesson to be learned here is that ninety percent of your diagnoses can be made by history. Talk to your patients, be thorough, and they will tell you what's wrong with them. You don't need labs, imaging studies, or technology if you talk to your patients and use your clinical skills. A thorough history by the intern on this case could have saved thousands of dollars and prevented any delay in the patient's treatment. Remember, your main purpose is to relieve suffering, prevent disability, and prolong life. Don't treat the chart; treat the patient. Don't rely solely on technology: evaluate the patient's clinical picture. Base your treatment on the patient, not an algorithm, don't follow a best practice guideline to change the treatment if the patient is improving. Best practice guidelines are good, but one size doesn't always fit all. Many patients improve despite our intervention, not because of it. Less is more in many cases, especially in elderly patients. Yes, you are dealing with a complex biological organism, but you are also dealing with a human being. Never leave the human factor out of the equation. The doctor-patient relationship is part of the healing process. Touch your patients, examine them, make physical contact, not only to aid in your diagnosis, but to connect with the patient. The laying on of hands has a healing effect and promotes trust in your patients. Patients who trust and rely on their doctors have better outcomes. Don't jump on every recent technology or treatment that comes along before it is thoroughly tested and proven. On the other hand, don't lag behind new advancements that can enhance your quality of care. Never be the first, never be the last, and your patient will never suffer because of you. But again, the lesson to be learned from this case is to talk to your patients, get to know them as human beings, not just as cases or diagnoses to be treated by an algorithm or by following best practice guidelines. Healing is an art as well as a science. Your interaction with your patients is a part of the art of healing. Always depend on your clinical skills and don't forget your humanity. Thank you for your time. Tomorrow, we will begin in earnest."

Tom and Jay were waiting for Dave and Henry at the door. "Do you guys want to catch some lunch before clinic? We have plenty of time."

Dave declined. "I'm going back to the station and go over all my patients again. I have no illusions; our convivial attending intends to be up my ass with spiked track shoes. In his eyes I'm far from excellent. I'm not a ten percenter, I'm a rotator, and I have low ambitions. He's going to make my life a living hell. I need to keep my head down, stay below his radar, and make sure he doesn't have any reason to come down on me."

"Don't overreact. Do a decent job for Sheffield and don't worry about him. I'm going to get lunch. I will bring you a sandwich and a Coke." But Henry knew Dave was right: they were all in for it, but Dave would catch the worst of it.

Dave ground his way through his patient's treatment plans and made notes about the things he needed to do on afternoon rounds. He rushed to the clinic, gobbled the ham sandwich, and chugged the Coke. The patients on his clinic schedule were hospital follow-ups or had chronic illnesses, so all he needed to do was check their labs and adjust their treatments. After clinic, he went back to the wards, made rounds, completed all the tasks in his notes, signed out to his counterpart on Team One, grabbed dinner, and was home by seven. He was physically exhausted and emotionally drained when he reached his apartment.

She was waiting for him at his door. "This is the first time I've seen you dressed up. You're really a very nice-looking man. No wonder you had all those little Florence Nightingales fluttered around you when you were a student." He was dressed in brown designer slacks, a blue button-down dress shirt, a solid brown silk tie, and brown cap-toe dress shoes. "You look so professional. I like it." She put her arms around his neck and kissed him.

When he felt her body pressed against his, smelled her perfume, and tasted her kiss, all the fatigue, stress, and mental duress of the day melted away. It no longer mattered that his service was too big. It was not important that he had four or five patients who would probably never leave the hospital in his lifetime. Who cares if his attending is one of the biggest assholes he has ever met? He has her to come home to.

"Was it bad?" She could feel the tenseness in his body as he held her.

"Worse."

"Tell me about it."

"Never."

"You need to talk about things and not keep them bottle them up inside you."

"Not with you. I have Henry and Mike. I want to leave that toxicity at the door when I'm with you. If you want to help, you can make a place for us where I can forget about the hospital, a fantasy bubble, our fantasy bubble. Now, I need a shower, because I am very grungy, and a beer; no, more than one beer, because I really need to unwind.' He unlocked the door, and they went inside.

"Is there anything else I can do to create a world away from the hospital, our fantasy bubble?" She went to the frig and got two beers.

"You bet. I will show you later." He took one of the beers and headed for the shower. *It's going to be all right, because no matter how bad it gets there, I have this to counter it here, and it doesn't get any better than this.*

When he finished showering, he joined her in one of the bean bags, and finally relaxed in the comfort of her arms. He was in the cocoon of his apartment, protected from the outside world, and wrapped in her softness. He was focused on her, nothing else, and nothing else mattered because he had the whole night with her.

They both woke with the alarm at six because she had an eight o'clock flight. Every fiber of his being wanted her, but he willed himself to shower, dress, kiss her goodbye, and go.

Henry was already on the station. "I'm surprised you're here on time since you were probably with Sharon again."

"It took all my self-discipline to walk out of my apartment this morning. She's so sweet, so gentle, and loving it's pure torture every time I leave her." Dave sat down at his desk.

"I hear you; she is something." Henry had a faraway look in his eyes before he continued. "The senior resident is here for oversight only. He sees the patients, reviews the charts, and writes notes; that's all. The service is Jay, you, and me. The good news is the attending makes sure we can handle things, then stops meeting with us until the students start. So, the quicker we get on top of things, the quicker we get rid of Finkel."

Dave concentrated on the four patients clogging up his service. The patient with heart failure was waiting to get on cardiology's list for a transplant or be moved to a skilled nursing facility for long-term care. The patient with liver failure and ascites was terminal. He would have to approach the family about his hospice care and a skilled nursing facility for him. That left the patient with cellulitis and the patient with terminal cancer.

Because of his moribund obesity, the cellulitis patient required total care as well as treatment for his stasis dermatitis and cellulitis. He was huge, smelled as bad as he looked, and resembled a beached whale as he lay in the oversized hospital bed. Since the care he required was all that was keeping him in the hospital, Dave asked Home Health Service to do an evaluation on him. They concluded with the proper equipment they could treat him at home. Dave dictated a note, wrote orders, discharged him, and arranged for an ambulance to transport him.

The terminal cancer patient was a single mother with metastatic cancer of the ovary whose husband left her with their two children when he found out she had cancer. Julie refused any morphine to ease her pain because she was afraid it would kill her in her weakened condition. She was desperately clinging to life to protect her children. Her sister was taking care of the children, but she didn't have the resources to care for them permanently, so when Julie died, the children would go into foster care, unless her husband could be found. She was willing herself to stay alive because she was in foster care as a child and was determined to keep her children from suffering the same fate. Bald from chemotherapy and so emaciated she resembled a concentration camp victim; she was tenaciously hanging on to life until her husband was located. Dave was so amazed by her courage and will power, he was determined to help her. There was nothing he could do for her medically, but he could help find her husband so she could die peacefully and without pain.

He met with Social Services. They had exhausted all their approaches, given up on finding the husband, and were setting the children up for foster care. Julie told him her husband was an oilfield worker, so was his father, and they often worked jobs together. Dave directed Social Services to look for the husband's father instead of the husband. They found the father's wife living in the city, and she told them her husband was in West Texas working on a drilling rig. Social Services called the number the wife gave them and got the husband's father. The father told them his son was in California working on a pipeline and gave them his number. It took all day, but by early evening, the husband was on his way back from California to take custody of his children.

Julie broke down in tears when Dave told her, then agreed to take some morphine to ease the pain if she could see her children first. The sister brought the children in, Julie talked to them about living with their father, said goodbye to them, and died shortly after the first dose of IV morphine. Dave pronounced her with mixed emotions. He had helped her keep her children out of foster care, helped her die painlessly and peacefully, but he knew the morphine killed her.

When he finished his day, he sat in his car for a while reflecting on what he had done. It didn't matter that he had solved the problem of the cellulitis patient, it did not matter he had sent other patients home with their illness resolved or controlled: for the first time he had written an order that took a human life. Granted it was not meant to kill her, but only to relieve her pain. Granted she was barely alive and probably gave up when she knew her children were safe, but it was still his hand that wrote the order. Not for the first time, and certainly not for the last time, Dave questioned the presence of a caring God.

He pulled himself together and drove home with a heavy heart. He had lost his first patient and it was by his own hand. He set out in his career to save lives, but now he had taken a life, and not only had he lost a patient, but he had lost a part of himself. He would help other patients die peacefully and painlessly in the future without any emotion because of this case. The experience changed him. He would write orders for morphine on future terminal patients without it touching him because the part of him it would have touched was gone. Dave grieved for his lost patient, but he also grieved for the lost part of himself. He knew there would be other cases that would affect him in some way that changed him. Once again, he asked himself if he wanted to make that kind of sacrifice. The question brought him back to the struggle of good versus evil and the realization that good is often consumed when confronting evil. Did he have the courage to be consumed to accomplish good? What bothered him most was wondering if he could even make a difference against the over-whelming mass of pathos in the human condition, or would he just be collateral damage?

He had given Sharon a key to his apartment, and she was waiting for him with all the candles burning and classical music playing. He felt as if he had a heavy overcoat on that contained everything he had dealt with that day in its pockets. He shrugged the coat off and left it on the ground as he crossed the threshold into his apartment, but unlike yesterday, he was different, and he could not shrug that difference off. When he saw her standing in front of him, that realization overcame him, and he pulled her to him. He held her without saying a word.

"Is the music OK or is it too sad? I thought you might need something soothing. Should I change it?" He was holding her so tight; she could hardly breathe.

"No. The music is perfect." He needed a lot to counter what he had dealt with today. He released her, went to the kitchen, got a beer, and poured Sharon a glass of wine.

She came to him in the kitchen. "Dave, I know what you said about not talking about your work, but don't lock me out. I don't need details, but I want to be included in things that affect you the way something is affecting you tonight. Talk to me. I want to help."

"It is nothing new. I don't know if I can do this, and what's more, I don't know if I want to do it. That's a hell of a realization after what I have been through to become a doctor. I thought I could use our world to counter what happens at the hospital, but things happen there that change you and become a part of you. Because they are a part of me, I can't leave them at the door." For some reason, he felt better after talking to her about his dilemma.

She took the beer and wine from him and sat them on the counter. "You must decide what to do about your career, but you need to think long and hard before you give up on your dream. You just started. Give it some time before you decide, and make sure it's not an emotional decision, but an objective one you have thought through carefully and completely." He felt the weight on his heart lift a little and joy seep back into his life as she put her arms around his neck. "Now go shower. I can see you need distracting tonight."

When he came out of the bathroom the music was still playing softly, it was dark, the curtains were closed, and the only light was the light from the candles. He smelled her perfume before he saw her silhouetted in the bedroom door. He picked her up and carried her to his bed. He lost himself in their lovemaking, slipping away from reality in the ecstasy he experienced every time they had sex. Afterwards, they fell asleep in each other's arms.

The next morning his adrenaline was up, but this time it was more than simply excitement, there was also an element of fear. He was amped up to be on call. Being on call in a big city, county teaching hospital required maximum effort. It was like being in the batter's box and you had to hit every pitch thrown at you.

Jay and Henry were waiting for him in the doctor's station when he arrived. "As the on-call team we're also the code team. Since this is our first call, I'll be the code leader, but in the future, whoever gets there first will be the code leader. We respond to codes on the medicine floors and codes in the common areas of the hospital, and by respond, I mean you run to the code site." Jay was amped up too.

Carol stuck her head in the door. "Good luck," She looked at Jay, "I'll see you tonight and we can have a cup of coffee." The day charge nurse followed her. "Remember, we're a team and the nursing staff is here to help you. Don't hesitate to call on us. If it gets crazy, and it does sometimes, we may get behind, but don't worry. We'll catch up."

Dave began his morning rounds. There were no rounds with the attending when they were on call, and by the time he went to rounds with the chief, he had everything under control. The amylase was down on his patient with pancreatitis, so he discharged him. The patient with pneumonia was afebrile for twenty-four hours and went home on oral antibiotics. The patient with liver failure was ready to go to a nursing home for hospice care, and Cardiology was had decided about the patient with cardiomyopathy. At lunch Dave asked Jay about Carol, "Is our boy Jay or Doctor McDonald having coffee with hot nurse Carol tonight?"

Jay blushed and fidgeted, "Ah, … Doctor McDonald. She's checking to see if I'm having trouble with you … with you and Henry. When I was on this service as an intern, I didn't … ah, get along with the other interns. She was nice to me and ah, … protected me. She wants to know if you guys are treating me … ah, you know, okay?"

Dave remembered what Sharon said about him being well dressed. Jay was a good guy and a good doctor. If he dressed better and took care of his appearance, it might make a difference in how people perceived him, and that could make a difference in how they treated him. "Jay, do you know about the dress code?"

"What dress code?" Jay looked up from his lunch.

"We can wear scrubs when we are on call. I am going to change after lunch. Do you ever wear scrubs when you're on call?" It looked as if Jay had slept in the clothes he had on.

"I don't like scrubs; they make me look too skinny." Jay looked troubled. He did not know where this conversation was going.

"Do you know what we are supposed to wear when we aren't on call?" Dave asked.

"A tie." Jay was definitely worried now.

"We are supposed to wear a dress shirt, tie, dress pants, and nice shoes. I think you would get less flak from people if you dressed better. Henry is going to give you a note to take to Bob and Phil's Clothing downtown. They'll help you buy some new clothes."

"I am?" Henry looked up from his lunch.

"I can't afford to buy clothes." Jay looked more than worried, he looked frightened.

"Take my advice and do this. Plus, get a good haircut, comb your hair, and start using some decent products."

"I cut my own hair." Jay looked from one of them to the other. He was totally off balance.

"Why am I not surprised? I think if you follow my advice, it will make a difference in the way people treat you."

Henry pulled out his notebook, tore out a page, scribbled on it, and gave it to Jay. "There is a good barber just down the street from the clothing store. Give this to one of the store owners, not a clerk or manager, but one of the owners. He will take care of you. I agree with Dave. Buy some clothes and get a haircut. If you do, Jay instead of Doctor McDonald, might end up having coffee with hot nurse carol when we're on call. She likes you."

Dave got his first admission around two o'clock that afternoon, and it was an easy one. The man was playing golf and had chest pains while walking the course. His EKG in the ER was normal as were his labs and his pain resolved with rest and oxygen. He was admitted for a cardiology work up and consult. He got four more admissions and finished a little after three in the morning.

Around mid-night he participated in his first code. They were sitting in the doctor's station when the code was called. "Code Blue, Medicine

One, room one eleven." Jay was out the door first with Dave and Henry right behind him. The Medicine One charge nurse was waiting for them with the crash cart when they got to the room.

The patient was in ventricular fibrillation, so Jay shocked him right away. He went back into sinus rhythm, and his vitals were stable by the time everyone on the code team got there. After the patient was transferred to the CCU, Jay stayed to write the transfer orders and note.

Walking back Henry asked Dave, "How did you learn to intubate like that? I turned my head and when I looked back, you already had him tubed even before Jay had a chance to shock him."

"I learned one night in the Medicine ER when I was a student. Mike and I were on together and a troll came in under CPR. We both tried to tube him but failed. The guy was found on the street, and no one knew how long he had been down, but since the EMTs had started CPR, the resident felt obligated to go through the motions. After he pronounced the patient, he told us we needed to learn how to intubate. He had us take the guy to the last bed in the back of the ER and tube him over and over until he was satisfied, we were proficient at intubation. The guy was a full-on troll who had been living under an overpass somewhere drinking wine, pissing and shitting himself for God knows how long. I never smelled anything so bad in my life. Mike threw up, and I know I threw up in my mouth a few times. His teeth were rotten, so we broke and dislodged some of them, then at one point we dislocated his jaw. We must have tubed him a hundred times. The resident came back from time to time to check our technique, but he made us keep at it all night. Mike was mad about it, but I realized the resident and interns were doing extra work so we could learn intubation. The next morning the resident told me a resident made him do the same thing when he was a student, and he thanked him mentally every time he had to intubate a patient. That experience taught me something besides how to intubate. It's not the old 'see one, do one, teach one' thing. It's about repetition and doing or seeing something over and over: like practicing a sport or a musical instrument. You have to do it, or see it, over and over, practicing until you get good at it. That's why we have to see so many patients. It's not about how much time we spend learning our craft: it's about the number of patients we see, practicing what we do over and over until we have perfected our abilities. It is not a time game; it's a numbers game. I just wish there was an easier way to go about it."

"You've changed in the last few days, Dave. You seem more mature. Are you finally growing up and joining the rest of us in the real world?" Henry's protective nature came out.

"I came to grips with things. I learned you need to give up a part of yourself and stop putting yourself first if you want to be a physician. I was afraid of giving up who I was, to become what I want to be, but I think I'm ready now."

After his last admission, he slept for a few hours, then got up to round on his patients and those signed out to him. He was dead on his feet by the time he got to his apartment. He called Sharon, "Hi, Baby. I'm home, and I'm going to sleep. I will see you at four."

The alarm went off at three and the only thing that kept him from turning it off and going back to sleep was knowing she was waiting for him. She answered the door dressed for the Fourth of July in white shorts, a red silk blouse, and a blue silk scarf tied at the side of her neck.

"Can we skip the picnic?" He reached for her.

"No, I spent a lot of time getting ready, and I'm not going to let you get me unready, yet. We are going to the picnic, the concert, the fireworks, and the party. I intend to enjoy myself with barbecue, music, fireworks, and dancing with a cute guy if he plays his cards right." She brushed past him but stopped at the door, "I was lonely last night. I've gotten used to sleeping with you and the bed felt empty without you. I know you're busy when you're on call, but I wish you would call me, if only to say good night."

"You bet." He took her hand, and they walked to the house next door.

When they arrived at the door, Phil and Bob were standing in the entryway with two women. "Gorgeous, you look radiant: you are positively glowing. Hi Dave, from the way my beautiful friend looks, I assume the good doctor's treatment is agreeing with her. Rachael and Sam, this is Dave. Dave, Rachael and Sam are our friends and like Bob and I, they are married."

"Is everyone here? Are we the last ones?" Sharon asked.

Phil looked around. "No, Sherry and Henry aren't here yet."

"Henry and I were on call last night, and I finished my last patient around three. I know he got one after me." Dave had barely finished talking when Sherry and Henry walked in.

"Hi, everyone, let's get this party started." Every man there was dressed like Dave in shorts, a T-shirt or polo shirt, and athletic shoes. All the women had followed the same motif as Sharon, shorts, a top, and sandals in a red, white, and blue color scheme. Not Henry, he had on khaki pants, a white dress shirt, and loafers without socks. That was as casual as Henry ever got for anything. Sherry was dressed in slacks, a blouse, and sandals.

"Are you okay, Henry? I know you got less sleep than I did." Henry looked like he had not slept at all.

"I am running on empty, but I am running, and I have enough fuel to last the rest of the day." Henry showed Dave a flask. "Most of us know each other, but since some of us don't, let's go around and everyone can introduce themselves. I am Henry, and this is my paramour, Sherry."

Sherry pushed Henry and laughed. There were twenty of them including Mike with his blind date Janice, Harvin and Connie an ICU nurse, George, and the graduate student he was dating plus Sharon's roommates, Audrey, and Jake a pilot, Caroline, and Ron a financial advisor, and Helen with her date. The girl with Mike was cute, but she was short and built like an adolescent boy. Pam, the woman with George was attractive but like George, withdrawn and quiet. The pilot looked like a pilot, handsome, rugged, and masculine. The financial advisor looked slick.

Sherry had taken care of everything with help from Haven and George. They had secured three tables on the edge of the open area in front of the stage and placed lawn chairs in front of the tables. Plastic plates, wine glasses, and flatware along with foil covered platters containing baked beans, coleslaw, potato salad, ribs, barbecued chicken, brisket, and cornbread were on each of the tables. Beer, white wine, and bottled water were in a cooler and there were bottles of red wine on the tables. Sherry considered this her party, and if it was her party, it was going to be done right.

"Haven and George brought a couple of Frisbees, a smash ball set, and a football over to play with. There is beer for the boys, wine for the ladies, and waters. The concert starts at eight and the fireworks are after sunset. Harvin set up some speakers in the front room, and we moved all the furniture to the walls to make room to dance after the fireworks."

Dave got a beer and was about to take a sip when a football flew at him. He caught it with his left hand and looked up to see who threw it.

"Sharon told me you played a little ball." The pilot was standing with Sharon and Audrey. "I was looking for someone to play catch with."

"As long as it doesn't interfere with my beer drinking." He took a sip of beer and threw the ball back. The pilot fired the ball back at Dave who caught it easily with one hand. They moved further apart and continued to throw the ball back and forth. The pilot began to bare down and cut loose with some fastballs, but Dave reached out and snagged them, took a sip of beer, and tossed the ball back.

"You have really soft hands." Jake said.

Dave added. "And you have a good arm. I take it you were a quarterback."

"How soft are his hands, Sharon?" Audrey asked and laughed.

Sharon walked over to Dave. "Why do grown men throw a funny-shaped pointy ball around to show how hard they can throw it or how easily they can catch it. I thought you were over all that." As she walked away with Audrey, she noticed Mike had abandoned Janice, and was lurking nearby watching her. Sharon was used to men looking at her, but Mike's stare made her uncomfortable. She quickened her pace to escape the dark pale of his attention and the cold shroud it cast over her. "Audrey, there's something wrong with that guy." She tilted her head toward Mike. "He's creepy and I don't understand why Dave hangs out with him."

Later they sat around talking, and Dave got to know Jake. He was in ROTC in college, went straight into the Air Force when he graduated, and served out his obligation to the military getting multi-engine time. When he got out, he applied to the airlines. He was in his late twenties, a little older than most of them, and he had decided he was going to ask Audrey to marry him as soon as he was sure she would say "yes". Audrey was practical, smart, and reliable, with the clean, Ivory Soap girl next door looks that All American hero types like Jake could not resist. They were the perfect wholesome Hallmark Couple.

The four flight attendants and their dates sat together. Henry and Sherry, Bob and Phil, Rachael and Sam sat at one table, while George and Pam, Mike and Janice, and Harvin and Connie sat at another table. Connie was a bright, pretty, well-endowed blonde in her early twenties. Today, her endowments were encased in a red top that displayed a portion of them and augmented them significantly, much to Harvin's delight. Connie was sitting next to Mike, and he could hardly take his eyes off her chest long enough to take a bite of food. She decided if he wanted to look, she would give him a good look, so she leaned over to get something in front of him and put the exposed portion of the contents of her top only inches from his nose.

Harvin admonished her. "Don't do that. I know what you're doing, and he will too."

Mike asked, "What did he say," and Connie replied, "He said he likes Georgia peaches, too" Connie was from Georgia.

"I don't get it." Janice did not get a lot of things.

George, who had been watching quietly, as he always did, made a comment, which he almost never did, "Harvin is partial to Georgia peaches." They all laughed except Janice and Mike.

"Where is the cafeteria monitor? The table over there is out of control, the table with the young ones, they're disturbing our dinner. Something needs to be done about those children; they're having too much fun." Henry threw a piece of cornbread at George.

"Act your age, Henry." Sherry smacked the hand that had thrown the cornbread. Henry threw another piece of cornbread at Harvin. "You are disturbing your elders. Stop having fun."

Mike knew he was the object of their laughter, and he was not happy about it, but it never occurred to him it had started with him staring at Connie's breasts. They finished eating, cleared everything away, dumped the garbage, moved to the chairs and some blankets the flight attendants brought, and faced the stage. While they were waiting for the concert, Dave talked to Ron, the financial advisor, with Caroline. A Princeton graduate with a degree in finance and an MBA; he was polite, well-mannered, and reserved. He was devoted to Caroline; who was breezy, outgoing, friendly, and fun loving; his exact opposite.

The city symphony set up on the stage with the university's color guard standing to one side and played the national anthem. The rest of the concert consisted of rousing patriotic songs and folk favorites like "America the Beautiful" and "This Land Is Your Land." After the concert, everyone repositioned their chairs and blankets to watch the fireworks that were going to be set off over the lake at the other end of the park. There were "oohs and aahs" as the rockets soared into the night sky, leaving a faint smoke trail, before exploding in bright, sparkling displays of glitter, or flashes of vividly colored splashes that rained down like large glowing rain drops.

After the fireworks, they returned to the house, and Harvin started the music. Every holiday there are multiple parties in the houses that line the park, and the young crowd who live on the park go from house to house enjoying a sort of mobile neighborhood block party. College students, graduate students, and young professionals began to wander in and out of the house. The crowd of people getting beer and wine in the dining room or dancing in the front room expanded and contracted as the party playlist played on.

Watching Sharon's dance had an erotically enchanting effect on Dave. The music pulsing through her triggered all her training and she entered a trance-like state as she became one with the driving beats and rhythmic baselines. It was sensual and beautiful. But Dave was not the only one fascinated by her dancing, so were several other men in the room, including Mike. He was enthralled and was unable to look away from her captivating movements.

It was close to twelve when it all ended with everyone swaying and singing along with, "Hold her, squeeze her, don't ever leave her, you gotta, you gotta, try a little tenderness." It was the perfect way to end the party and the day. The police had started going around shutting down the house parties, so flashing red lights appeared on the street, and a police officer came to the door. Sherry was way more than buzzed, but she tottered over to talk to him. "Is it night-night time?"

The police officer scowled at her, "Yes, and I hope everyone at this party lives here, or near here, because if we see anyone from this party get in a car, they are going straight to jail."

She turned to the group. "The nice policeman said it's night-night time, so say goodnight and go find a place to sleep," she giggled, "... or whatever." She turned back to him and smiled, "We'll be good. I promise."

The police officer frowned, "Lady, you need to get to bed." Sherry giggled again, then called to Henry, "Henry, the nice policeman said you have to take me to bed now."

A week after the party, Sharon was alone in the house, her room-mates were out and Dave was at the hospital, when Mike walked in. It was late, she was downstairs making sure the doors were locked, when he walked in without ringing the bell. "Hi, Sharon."

"Mike! Dave's not here," She was dressed for bed in a skimpy, sheer nighty, "and I'm not dressed."

"I didn't come to see Dave, I came to see you, and you're dressed perfectly for why I came." He flashed her a sly smile.

"Why are you here Mike?" She realized he had been drinking.

"Dave's at the hospital so I thought you might be lonely and need some company?" He moved close to her.

"Forget it, Mike. Dave and I are exclusive."

"Dave's not the exclusive type. He always had more than one woman keeping his bed warm when we lived together. Don't you need more than one man keeping yours warm?" There was an overwhelming hunger in his eyes as he looked at her body through the flimsy material of the nighty.

"No Mike, I don't sleep around, and I'm with Dave. We're a couple. You need to leave, and I need to get to bed. I have an early trip tomorrow." She knew she had to maintain control. The slightest hesitation or sign of weakness, and he would be all over her with nothing to protect her but a scant scrap of transparent cloth.

"I heard you dated a lot of different guys and I saw what happened with Dave. You want me to believe you only hook up with him now. I okay with getting to bed any time you're ready." He was becoming aroused looking at her in the short sexy nighty, and his voice dripped with lust as he moved up against her.

She walked confidently around him and opened the door. "Leave, Mike. I'm going to bed now and I'm going alone. I not going to sleep with you, so leave." She held the door open and stood behind it, using the door to shield her body from the longing in his eyes.

"A woman as hot as you screwing only one guy? I don't believe it. I've watched you. You're way too sexy for that." He walked toward her again.

She moved further behind the door. "Believe it Mike; believe it and leave, but I'll tell you if that changes." The disappointment was visible in his face, but by giving him hope, she also was giving him a reason to leave. "You'll definitely be the first man I will tell when I'm dating again. Now, please leave." He was too drunk to notice the sarcasm in her voice.

"You'll hook up with me when Dave's gone?" Hope replaced the disappointment on his face.

"Yes." She pointed him out the door, unaware she had planted a festering seed that would continue to grow even without being nurtured. She locked the door, turned, leaned against it, took a deep breath, and tried to calm her racing heart.

For the next two months Sharon bid her trips around Dave's schedule. She did not tell him about Mike's late-night visit. It had nothing to do with him and she did not want to create a problem that could spill over to the hospital. She handled Mike and defused the situation by putting Dave up as a barrier; all she needed to do now was avoid Mike, and eventually he would go away. She had dealt with men like him at work and she knew how to handle them.

When Dave was on call, she bid on layovers, and she bid on turn-arounds for the nights they spent at his apartment. On his call nights, Dave called to tell her good night, and talk for a while. The nurses listened and began to ask from the nurse's station, "How is Baby tonight?" They were touched by the snippets of the conversations they heard from his side, and he began to find coffee waiting for him on his desk every morning, and his charts pulled up. Henry asked Jane about it, and she told him the nurses had developed a soft spot for Dave and Baby.

Finkel tormented them for a couple of weeks after the Fourth, then he stopped showing up, but rounds with Sheffield became more intense each time they were on call. He would use his favorite admonishments, "You can't not know that!", "You can't make that kind of mistake!", "When you make a mistake, your patient suffers, not you!", "You are here for your patient, to relieve their pain and suffering, and to prevent their disability and death.", "stay focused on your patient!" God help any intern who let the patient's potassium fall or overshot their blood sugar treating their diabetes. Oxygen saturations not maintained in pulmonary patients led to tirades. Rounds with the chief were brutal but fair, and Sheffield handed out praise as well as criticism. He constantly taught, motivated, and encouraged during rounds with the chief.

Dave admitted a hundred and twenty patients to the Medicine wards, and he became proficient at treating most of the common ailments that led to hospitalization. He also managed a litany of chronic and acute illnesses in over six hundred clinic visits he did. With his clinic visits, rounds, and admits, he had close to fifteen hundred patient contacts during his first two months as an intern. His confidence and ability, along with his clinical skills, grew day by day as he ground through the work.

There were multiple cases that affected him psychologically, and each one left its mark on him, but each one helped prepare him to handle emotionally challenging cases better the next time he encountered one. He had trouble maintaining his weight and he was always tired by the end of his rotation. Sharon did everything she could to help, but his coping mechanisms were barely keeping him functional. There were always at least ten to twelve extremely ill patients on his list, and there was no respite because he was responsible for them seven days a week. He was always worried, anxious, and constantly feared he may have missed something or failed to do something for one of his patients.

He was in the hospital working with hardly any sleep for thirty-six hours during his on-call day and the day after call, then he was back for another twelve hours on the third day unless it was a weekend. There were times it was worse. He admitted an alcoholic type-one diabetic who had been on a bender, drinking nonstop for a week. At first, he did not think she was going to survive because her sugars were off the charts, she was profoundly ketonic, and her renal function, liver functions, and electrolytes were all grossly abnormal. He was up with her all night, reviewing her labs every hour and adjusting her treatment. Sheffield looked at her chart the next day and simply shook his head without saying a word. He was with her all day, even though he had clinic that afternoon. Finally, she came under control late that night. He was at the hospital working with no sleep or rest for two days by the time he signed out to the on-call intern and left for his apartment, but he had to be back at the hospital the next morning. Sheffield had been right, the medicine Wards tested him to his very core, but they had also prepared him to be a doctor.

Chapter 3

Sharon

Dave was not on call on the last weekend of his rotation on the wards, and he wanted to go out to celebrate. They had not gone out since the party on the Fourth of July, so they made plans with Audrey and Jake to go to Mother's Blues, a popular club in the city, and she wanted something new to wear. He skipped Grand Rounds and picked her up at house well before noon on Saturday morning.

Bob and Phil's Clothing for Discerning Men and Women was surrounded by the most exclusive stores, shops, and eateries in the city. Sharon led Dave to the women's department, picked out a couple of dresses, and had the salesclerk take her to one of the dressing rooms. As soon as the clerk left, he was in the dressing room. "You're not supposed to be in here." He reached for her. "Don't even think about it. I see the look in your eyes. Go wait for me in the fitting room. Jesus, you're so difficult." He trapped her against the wall with one arm on each side of her.

"Behave, you're like an unruly child." She tried to wiggle free, but he wrapped his arms around her and pulled her to him. "I can't help it, I haven't seen you for two days, and I have to molest you a little."

They heard a woman's voice. "Is there a man in there? I hear a man's voice."

She pushed him away and put her finger to her lips.

"I'm going to get a manager. There aren't supposed to be any men in the women's dressing rooms."

"Get out." She pushed him out the door, quickly slipped on one of the dresses, and joined him in the fitting room.

"Why am I not surprised it's you two?" They saw Phil standing in the door of the fitting room with a woman behind him. "Don't worry,

64

Mrs. Roberts, I will take it from here." He dismissed the woman, "Were you really going to do it in one of my dressing rooms?"

"Phil! I'm trying on dresses. We're going clubbing tonight and I want something new to wear." She looked hurt and pouted a little for him.

"You are a terrible liar, Gorgeous. And you Dave, I told you to cherish her; not to bang her in public." Phil shook his head and laughed. "It's almost noon. Find something you like, and I will take you two to lunch."

"Do you like this dress, Phil? Do you like it, Dave?" She posed with her hands on her hips.

"I like it, but I want to see the others. Sit down Phil." Dave patted the seat of the chair next to him. "Help her pick something."

"What the hell, I have nothing better to do, like run a store, so I might as well waste time with you two. Maybe I can keep you out of trouble." Phil sat down.

After she tried on the other dresses, she asked them, "Which one?"

Dave said, "The first one."

"She makes everything she puts on look good, but I agree, the first one." Phil took the dress, pressed a button on the wall, and the salesclerk appeared. "Take this dress, ring it up as a no-charge, then call Andre's and get me a table for three."

Sharon protested, "You can't do that, Phil. That is an expensive dress and Andre's for lunch."

"It's my store, I can do what I want, and that's where I want to go for lunch. Come on. We can walk." Outside, Phil held Dave's arm to let Sharon walk ahead. "What have you done to her? It's like she's a different person."

"She's done something to me too, Phil. I've never been happier."

She came back to them. "Why are you guys lagging? What are you talking about?"

Phil responded. "He said you make him happy, now let's eat." He opened the door to Andre's.

They lingered all afternoon in Andre's. Phil told Dave about Stonewall and the difficult fight the gay community waged and is still wagging to secure their rights. Dave's respect and admiration for Phil grew as the afternoon morphed into the longer shadows of the ending of the day. He was not only Sharon's friend, but he was also her confidant, her advisor, and she depended on him for support: he was basically a father figure to her.

Later when they were alone, she told him. "I'm happy too. I'm happier than I've been for a long time, but this has all happened so fast. Is it even real or is my happiness some fabricated fantasy? We have been together almost constantly since the night we met. The other people in my life, like you, have faded into the background, and my whole existence revolves around him: him and the incredible sex we have every time we're together. Is that it? Are we simply two moths drawn to, and circling a bright flame, the white-hot flame of sex, or is it genuine and there's more to it?"

Back at her house, she took the dress with her to the bathroom. "I don't want you to see me until I'm ready. Jesus, did I just objectify myself."

She came out of the bathroom, turned with her arms out, and modeled the dress for him. "You look magnificent." He slid his arm around her waist, took her hand as she put her other arm over his shoulder, and they waltzed around the room to no music, until he stopped, held her, and kissed her. She put her arms around his neck and returned his kiss, then pushed him away reluctantly. "We have to go. Jake will be here any minute. We'll finish this later." She rotated out of his arms and danced away from him.

Mother's Blues was in an Afro-American community, but it catered to the students from the university, and the young professional crowd that lived in or near the city. After they found a table and ordered drinks, Sharon pulled Dave onto the dance floor, and they danced until the band took a break. He pulled her to him. "I love to watch you dance."

She wrapped her arms around his neck, hooked one leg behind his knees, and kissed him. Her hair was down around her face, her skin was glowing, and she was glistening with sweat. She whispered, "You know what dancing is don't you? It's foreplay."

They were dancing next to a Black couple and the man put his arm around his partner as he looked at Sharon. "She sure can move, but she's running hot. She's got the fever. You better take her home and treat it right away."

She threw her head back and laughed. "I think he's right."

"Like I said, you better get her home, put her to bed, and treat that fever." He pulled his partner closer. "It looks like it's getting worse, but if you like to dance, and it sure looks like she does; this is the place. Maybe we'll see you here again." The woman nodded to Sharon. The man held his fist out and Dave fist bumped him.

They returned to the park as the full moon was just beginning to peek the very top of its snowy white head, above the trees. Sharon put her arms around Dave's neck and leaned back. "Best day ever."

"Really?" He looked at her lovely face with the light of the moon on it.

"Yes, I feel free to be who I am when I'm with you. It's hard to explain. We can talk about it tomorrow, but now I want to take advantage of all that foreplay. Like the man said, I've got the fever, and you need to treat it right away, doctor." They followed Audrey and Jake to the house, but she stopped at the door. "I want you to make love to me outside in the soft grass under the full moon."

She got a blanket, they found a secluded spot on the lawn behind the house, and there in the moonlight, under the stars, he took her to a mindless state where she was unaware of anything other than the exquisitely intense pleasure pulsing through her body. Later, their mindless passion spent, they moon bathed and talked.

Sharon told him how she was bullied as a child. "My eyes caused me a lot of pain when I was younger. The doctor said I have a mutation that caused the cells in my irises to fail to produce enough pigment. There is green pigment around the edges but not much in the body of the iris itself. My skin is light too, so people thought I was an albino. Children can be so cruel. They made fun of me, called me names, and wouldn't play with me, but the adults were worse. Some of them told their children my eyes were the mark of the devil. Others said I was a witch, and they wouldn't let their kids near me. I'm sure I would have been burned at the stake in an earlier century. When I matured, the same boys who tormented me couldn't stay away from me. I was everything in high school: homecoming queen, prom queen, most beautiful, top of my class. The boys I grew up with acted as if I would simply shine on what they did to me, but I didn't. I gravitated to others who were bullied and knew what it felt like. They were gentle and kind, I felt safe with them. I was nice to everyone, but I didn't get involved with the popular crowd." The girls were jealous of me, and the boys wanted to screw me.

She didn't tell him about her father, or how she felt about marriage and children, she might eventually, but not now. Her current life was the product of her past experiences: her previous interactions with men, her childhood traumas, and her parents' troubled divorce. She didn't tell him any more about Bar either, because her relationship with Bar had left an indelible imprint on her psyche. She was ashamed and embarrassed by what happened with him, and now he was trying to get back into her life.

Since she told him about her eyes, he thought he should tell her about his sister. "I had a sister. She was born with severe birth defects that weren't compatible with life, but she lived for two years. I went to her room every day." He had to stop and compose himself. "She had a pretty face but the rest of her was hard to look at. I was a child so I couldn't understand why God would do something like that to a baby. She was an innocent baby. Why did she have to suffer?" He almost broke down. "My sister's death broke my mother's spirit. I don't know how she had the courage to have another child, but my parents wanted the standard two children, a boy, and a girl. My mother desperately wanted a girl with her last pregnancy, but she got my brother instead."

He went on to the worst part. "My sister's death hit me hard. After the funeral, I still went to her room every day, but she wasn't there. Where was she? What was death? I didn't understand it and I still don't. I became a doctor because I want to prevent suffering, but most of all, I want to prevent death."

She had no idea he was so vulnerable and hid so much emotion, or that he had a tormented soul that drove him to help others in order to ease his own pain. His life had been shaped by his sister's birth and death. He was compelled to be a doctor; there was no other choice for him, no matter how insecure or troubled he was by his training, he had to become a physician.

They viewed events in their lives through a lens to their past. That lens programmed their brains to form a paradigm they used to evaluate and analyze the present. They both had experienced childhood traumas, by sharing those traumas they developed a better understanding of themselves, they became more comfortable with each other, and they felt that they were not alone anymore.

They moon bathed in the subdued light and enjoyed the touch of their intertwined bodies as they explored each other's enter most selves. A unique bond formed between them as they lay on the blanket in the soft grass caressed by the warm night air in the soft glow of the full moon. A bond that was destined to grow into something more

The next morning after rounds, they went to the park, found a bench, and sat down. "There's a reason I'm struggling with my internship. It's not only the fatigue, the long hours, and the sleep deprivation. I see things no one should see, and I can't unsee them; I hear things no one should hear, and I can't unhear them; I'm exposed to things no one should be exposed to, and it all affects me. The beauty and sweet music of my life is blotted out by the darkness of the pathos of the human condition I encounter daily at the hospital." Dave shifted his position on the bench to face her.

"Let me give you an example. I will tell you about one case, not just the medical part, but the whole story we pieced together from the EMTs, the police, and her girlfriends; then we are never going to talk about what I do again. I don't want to bring that toxicity in our time together." Sharon nodded.

"I did a neurosurgery elective my senior year, not because I was interested in neurosurgery, but because I could do it at DG in Denver and ski. We admitted a gunshot wound to the head. She was eighteen years old, just old enough to work in a club, with a drug-dealing older boyfriend who hooked her on heroin. She worked every night at the club, gave him all her money, and he kept her strung-out on heroin. He wanted more money out of her, so he tried to turn her out to do tricks, and when she refused to prostitute herself, he beat her, cut her heroin off, and threw her out. Her friends said she suffered terribly from withdrawal symptoms, and when she couldn't take it any longer, she got a gun, went out in the alley behind the club, and shot herself." Sharon looked horrified. "She put the gun to her temple and pulled the trigger, but it was aimed too low and too far forward, so it just blew out her eyes." She gasped.

"This is too much for you." But she demanded he finish. "You've told me too much. I have to know it all."

"We operated on her, debrided the wounds and did some bone grafting, but spinal fluid continued to leak from the wound. She had to have a spinal tap every day to remove all her spinal fluid to relieve the pressure on the meninges, the coverings of the neural tissue, so they would heal. That's where I came in. I was the only student on the service, so I had to do a spinal tap on her every day. Not only did I have to tap her every day, but I also had to change her dressings and look into those two cavities in her face where her eyes used to be. She wanted to die. She screamed, pulled out her IVs, tore at her bandages, and had to be put in four-point restraints, but she still thrashed around and fought the restraints.

We tried to keep her sedated, but she would come out of it, and start screaming and fighting the restraints. I can still hear those screams and the awful sounds she made. The nurses had to hold her in position for the spinal taps, and even though she was sedated, she was still awake. I was a student, so it would take me a couple of attempts to get in: all while she was fighting, screaming, and making those awful sounds the whole time. By the time I finished, I would be shaking and covered with sweat. She hated the taps, and she hated me. She started screaming every morning when I got there.

The EMTs said they found blood trails in the alley where she crawled around trying to find the gun to finish it and the shrink told me she would kill herself the first chance she got. The women she worked with said she was pretty and extremely popular with the customers at the club. Well, she wasn't that pretty now, and one of the things that got me was the way the staff talked about her. She was just a junkie whore. They made fun of her, said she was a one-bagger, and laughed about it. She was someone's baby girl. My mother would have given anything to have had a daughter.

I could've given her fifty milligrams of potassium IV, but even having a thought like that scared the hell out of me. What do you do with a thought like that? What do you do with something that makes you have a thought like that? They tell you to compartmentalize it, to put it in a box, and store the box away. I thought about taking her life. How do you put that in a box? How do you store a thought like that away? I can still see her, see the room, hear her screams, and smell the old dressings.

That was just one case during my clerkship in med school. How many cases like that does it take until you wall off your humanity and lose your empathy for the plight of others? How long before you lose yourself and who you are, trying to cope with a side of life no one should be exposed to? But you have to be trained and properly trained, you have to be the doctor in charge, you need to be in a city, county hospital where you're exposed to everything, and in a good program, where you're taught how to deal with everything you're exposed to."

"Didn't you have anyone you could talk to? Don't they provide some type of therapy to help you deal with experiences like that? No one should be expected to cope with that kind of horror without some sort of support." Sharon was incredulous.

"Not where I went to school. But you're right, sometimes I want to do a Joseph Conrad and scream, 'the horror, the horror.' I deal with it by distracting myself when I'm not at the hospital." He put his head down.

"I understand." She put her arms around his neck.

He looked up. "I'm sorry, you didn't need to hear that. You don't need to know things like that even exist. They aren't a part of your world, but they're a part of my world, and I wanted you to understand." *I will never let you see my world again. When we are together, we will stay in a world that suits you. A world where I can escape from the realities of my world and find refuge.* "Let's go to my place, spend the rest of the day at the pool, listen to some music, and get into some distracting later tonight. You will be gone on a layover tomorrow night and I will be on call when you get back, this could be the last night we have together for a while."

"OK, but no distracting in the morning. I have two long hard days ahead of me, and I have to be at the airport early. I can't be late because you can get fired for being late or missing a trip."

It was a sunny summer Sunday in a single's apartment in a large Southern city, so the pool was crowded. He pulled two lounge chairs close to a table with an umbrella to give them some shade and sat down. She took her cover-up off and lay down next to him. "Time for sunblock. I can already feel the burn." He relished applying sunblock to her body and it was a ritualistic behavior he reveled in each time they went to the pool.

"It's too hot. Let's go for a swim." She left him sitting there and walked confidently to the diving board, looked back, tossed her hair, walked forward, hit the diving board, and made a perfect dive with hardly a ripple. She came up treading water and he dove in to join her. "Where did you learn to dive like that?"

She put her arms around his neck, her legs around his waist, and made him tread water for the both of them. "There are clubs that have pools, golf courses, tennis courts, and places to eat that some families belong to."

He let them sink, and they swam to the shallow end of the pool where they could stand up. "So, you're a country club brat."

She looked a little sad, then brightened. "Until I went to college, but look who's talking, frat rat." She locked her arms and legs around him again. "I'm a barnacle stuck to a frat rat."

"Spoiled country club brats who are stuck-up sorority girls don't get to call fraternity men frat rats unless they can breathe under water." He went under with her wrapped around him.

She came up for air. "If you drown me, I won't be able to distract you later." He swam to the ladder, climbed out, and waited for her. She climbed partially out, stood on the ladder, and put her head back in the water to let her long hair stream down her back.

It began when he first saw her, grew as they got to know each other, accelerated with the sex, expanded exponentially last night, and now it exploded in him with an overwhelming force. *I think I'm in love with her.*

Sharon looked at him as she stood on the ladder. "What?" When he did not answer, she looked down at herself. "What? Am I coming out of my bikini?" She climbed out of the pool, adjusted her top, and walked up to him. He picked up a towel and wrapped it around her. "What? Did all that sunblock slathering and pool frolicking get you all worked up? I have on two layers of sunblock with no burn, and I am having fun, so you'll just have to cool your engines."

"That's not it. Well, it is in a way. I love you, Sharon. I know we've only known each other for a couple of months, but I think I'm in love with you."

"I might be in love with you too, Dave. You're right, we haven't known each other for a long time, so I'm not sure, but I feel something. I've never been in love before, so I don't know what it feels like, but I think what I feel for you could be love, or something that could turn into love." He crushed her to him, kissed her, and held her as he allowed what had just happened to sink in.

She pulled away, "People are watching. Wait until we go in." When they were back on their lounge chairs, she took his hand. "When we go in, I need to tell you some things." They spent the rest of the afternoon in the pool immersed in the joy of their newly expressed feelings for each other.

Back in the apartment, he grabbed her and fell into one of the beanbags. "Does this mean you need distracting now?" She maneuvered so they were face to face, smiled, and touched his lips with her fingertip. "I need to tell you some things first. You need to know I am never going to marry or have children. I want you to know that before we go any further with this relationship."

She searched his face. "You deserve to know why. My dad is a lawyer, my mom is a stay-at-home mom who never worked, and I am an only child. My dad is exceptionally good looking. My mom is pretty, but I get my looks from my dad. He makes a lot of money as a corporate lawyer and we had it all: the country club, nice cars, nice house, and I had anything I wanted. You're right, I was spoiled until college. It started when I was about sixteen. He cheated on my mom. She caught him time after time, but he kept seeing other women. It went on until I started college, then they got a divorce in my first year. They had been married for twenty years and my mom had no way of supporting herself, but my dad didn't want to give her any money. They fought in court for another year. Being a lawyer, he knew all the tricks.

When I was eighteen, he stopped paying child support, and managed to decrease what he was paying my mom to the bare minimum. My mom paid for my college, the sorority, and saw that I had what I needed on the support he paid her and the settlement. I worked in the summer and tutored during the school year, but I know she sacrificed for me. I haven't seen or spoken to my father since the divorce. I saw firsthand what can happen with marriage. I'm never giving up my name and my freedom by signing a contract to tie me to someone who can abandon me and take everything from me. He took everything I had from me, including having a father."

"I'm fine with whatever type of relationship you want, Sharon." He responded seriously.

She smiled mischievously at him. "Why, because I'm a good lay, Dr. Cameron? Is that all you're after?"

He laughed and went after the strings of her bikini. "I don't know. Let's see. Dirty talk is cheap. I judge performance."

Later, as they lay on the floor side by side with evening creeping in on them through the glass doors of the balcony, she confided in him, "I know you have been with a lot of girls, but I don't want to think about that. I don't want to think about you doing what we do with anyone else but me. I want to think I am the only girl you have ever been with, but you didn't learn how to do what you do on your own, and I don't think it was divine inspiration. Other women taught you and although I don't want to admit it, in a way I am grateful to them."

He turned on his side, rested on his elbow, and lightly ran his hand over her body. "You're right, there were some very hedonistic, plea-sure-seeking women focused on their own gratification who taught me a lot. Plus, I am a doctor, I know about the lady parts and what to do with them. We had a class on human sexuality in med school. But I learned that sex simply for pleasure, is a form of pornography; sex with someone you connect with is much better; and now I know making love is the most wonderful thing in the world. I must admit

I had a wonderful time learning, but it all comes together in making love to you." He laughed.

She rolled toward him and pushed his hand away. "You can be such an asshole. Don't touch me. I told you thinking about you with other women upsets me, then you give me a blow-by-blow account. You are cut off until further notice. I have to get the picture of you enjoying your lessons with your teachers out of my head before I let you touch me again."

He reached out and tried to pull her to him, but she wiggled free. "No, not until you learn how not to be hurtful."

He lay back with his hands behind his head. "OK, tell me about Bar. I told you about the women I have been with. Tell me about Bar."

She sat up. "No."

"Come on, I don't have any secrets from you. Tell me about Bar."

"There's nothing to tell. We were together and now we're not. It's in the past, so forget it. I have to forget God knows how many girls you've been with; you can forget the one guy I was with. Drop it." She lay back down beside him.

Lying in bed with him later that night she thought about the incident with Mike. Mike was creepy but Bar was dangerous, and his family is even more dangerous. Maybe she should tell Dave what happened with him, especially with what was happening lately. He probably needs to know in case Bar finds out about him or shows up.

She sat up in bed, locked her arms around her knees, and hugged them to her. "I'll tell you about Bar, but you have to promise that no matter what I say, you'll let it go."

He sat up beside her. "I promise."

She put her head down on her knees. "He hit me."

"I'll find him and pound his ass to a bloody pulp."

She replied. "No, you won't. You promised. I knew you would react this way. That's why I didn't want to tell you."

He held her by her shoulders and looked into her eyes. "Why do you want to protect someone who hit you and abused you? Understand, if anyone hurts you, I will go after them, and God help them when I get my hands on them." The storm she saw in his eyes was frightening, and she knew if that storm ever broke on someone, they would need God's help. She shrugged his hands off and put her arms around his neck. "His family is immensely powerful in this state. His father is known for his underhanded ruthless tactics and dirty politics. He wins elections by destroying his opponents. He would never allow anyone to hurt his golden child. He would retaliate. I can't allow anything to happen to you because of me. I'm protecting you, not him. You have no idea who these people are, how they operate, or how much power they have. Let it go. Keep your promise for your, sake not for his." He was silent. He was so angry, he couldn't speak. Regardless of what he promised or what she said about Bar's family, he knew he would unleash that anger on him if he ever had the opportunity.

"Let me tell you about it." She pulled him back down with her. "If I tell you about it, maybe we can both put it behind us. I need to start from the beginning for you to understand. Let me tell you about myself first. I didn't lose my virginity until I was in college. I had been dating this guy for a while, and I thought it was time, so I let him do it. Neither of us knew what we were doing, so there wasn't much to it. I certainly didn't get anything out of it. You're right, I get hit on all the time, especially on the plane, not just by the crew members, but by the passengers too, especially in first class. We're not supposed to date passengers, but everybody does. The first time I worked first class, a celebrity on the flight asked me out. He was incredibly good looking, charming, and polished. I was flattered and gave him my number. He called me after we landed and arranged to pick me up later that night. He didn't even come to the door: he sent his limo driver to get me. Once I was in the limo, he opened his pants and pushed my head down on him. I was young, naive, and starstruck, so I let him have his way with me. The driver drove us straight to his hotel. Once we were in his room, he took my clothes off, guided me to the bed, and pounded me as hard as he could, for as long as he could, until he was satisfied. He did me two more times, and when he was finally finished with me, he called the limo driver to take me home. The driver didn't even walk me to my door. He let me out on the street; sore, used, and humiliated, but I had learned my lesson. I would never make that kind of mistake again. The other men I dated after that want to hook up with me too, but like him, that's all they want. They just want to use me. I saw no reason to let someone use me for their own gratification and pleasure, especially when there was nothing in it for me."

She sat up again. "I have had sex with three men and to tell the truth, not that many times. You have been with a lot of women and had sex with them I don't know how many times. I don't want to think about how many women you have been with or how many times you've had sex with them, but I am supposed to be fine with it because you are a man. If a man has a lot of women, he is a stud, but if a woman has a lot of guys, she is a slut. That stupid double standard is why I was so worried about what you would think of me the night we met."

He sat up beside her. "Thinking about you with someone else drives me crazy." He was incredibly jealous of no one in particular and everyone in general.

She straightened up and looked at him. "Ditto, Dave, and I have a lot more to think about than you do." She settled back with her arms around her knees and continued. "So, I dated a lot of guys, but I said good night at the door. I was having a wonderful time: some guy took me out to dinner almost every night. Then last Summer, the med students moved in next door, and they came over right away to introduce themselves. Bar pursued me relentlessly until I finally went out with him."

She straightened up again and touched his lips with her fingertip. "Listen now, don't say anything, just listen, and when I am finished, it's over, never to be spoken of again, you won't do anything about it and we'll both forget it."

He nodded, but he knew what he would do to Bar if he ever met him. "Everything was great at first and I thought I had found the perfect man. He is the smartest person I have ever known; he's extremely well educated, very well mannered, exceedingly gracious, and amazingly charming. His father was governor then, and he took me around showing me off to all the people in his father's political circle, and I got caught up in the glamour. Bar and I didn't have sex that often and when we did, it was nothing like what we do. Before I met you, I thought sex was just for the guy, and the girl's only purpose was to satisfy the guy." Dave started to say something, but Sharon put her fingertip to his lips.

"Then he started putting me down in front of our friends, never in front of his parents, their friends, or anyone he knew through his parents, but in front of his med school buddies, and the people I knew. I got tired of it and told him I was through with him. He told me I couldn't leave him because I belonged to him. I told him I didn't belong to anyone, and he hit me hard in the face with his fist. It hurt like hell. He is a wimp, but it still left a red mark and a bruise later. After he hit me, he threatened me. He said I could never leave him. I was his, and no one else could ever have me. I called the police, but when the DA found out his father was the governor, he refused to prosecute him. He kept calling and coming over, but I didn't answer his calls and I kept the doors locked until he left for Boston." She didn't tell him that Bar knocked her down when he hit her, and as she cowered, crouched on the floor covering her head with her arms, he grabbed one of her arms, pulled it away, then repeatedly slapped her, screaming at her the whole time.

She also didn't mention the stalking, the repeated poundings on the front door in the middle of the night, or the threatening messages he left on her phone. Nor did she tell him about the calls from Boston that led to her deciding to tell him what happened. Bar called her and left messages telling her he would be back for her, and she had better be ready to go with him when he came for her. He left messages telling her he knew she wasn't flying and to pick up. How did he know she wasn't flying? Did he have a copy of her schedule? How did he get a copy of her schedule? She didn't tell Dave he left a message with his vacation dates, telling her to put in for a transfer, and to be ready to go with him when he came for her. She didn't tell him the whole story because she couldn't, it was too painful and too humiliating. She couldn't say it out loud, and definitely not to Dave.

Dave put his arms around her. She always felt safe in his arms, she had since the first time he put them around her the night they met, and they made her feel safe now. She knew he would protect her from Bar, but she was afraid if he had to, it could end badly for him.

Chapter 4

The Medicine ER

D ave was light-hearted when he entered the apartment because his responsibilities on the Medicine wards ended when he walked out of the hospital that night. He grabbed Sharon, lifted her up, and spun around the apartment, "I am free, 'thank God almighty, I'm free at last'. I want to go skinny dipping." He sat her down and began taking his clothes off.

She watched him undress with her hands on her hips. "I'm not going skinny dipping in an apartment pool, so forget it."

"If we can't go skinny dipping, then my apartment is clothing optional." He chased her to the bedroom where she relented, pulled off her T-shirt and stepped out of her shorts, but left her thong on. "Can't I leave it on? It leaves something to the imagination."

"No, that's not an option in my clothing optional apartment. I have a terrible imagination. I need the real thing."

"Fine." She wiggled out of the thong and lay on the bed with one arm over her head.

Dave lay down beside her. "I want to bask in your loveliness."

"Bask in my loveliness? You really have a tough time keeping that Southern charm in check, don't you? Bask away." She laughed and put both arms over her head.

He got up and pulled her up with him. "I want a nude beer and some nude music. Then I want to bask in you."

"I knew we would get around to that sooner rather than later." She smiled and followed him to the kitchen where he got a beer and poured her a glass of wine. He lit all the candles, turned off the lights, closed the curtains, and turned on the sound system; then he pulled her into a bean bag enfolding her in his arms as Etta James's hauntingly distinctive voice took control of their emotions. "At last, my love has come along", prompted a passionate kiss that was prolonged by the music until the song ended.

He untangled himself from Sharon, stood up and held out his hand as the strains of Hoagy Carmichael's masterpiece, "Stardust" filled the apartment. He whispered in her ear, "That's all we are you know, just stardust. We are a unique collection of stardust that miraculously ignites into life. We're the stuff of stars forged in their nuclear furnaces before they explode in spectacular supernovas scattering their contents across the cosmos." As they slow danced around the room, their nude bodies pressed together, enveloped in the scent of the candles, it was difficult for him to imagine that the warm wave of pleasure surging through his body created by Sharon's soft form being enfolded in his arms could be connected to elements of the universe or science.

Etta James surprised her although she knew he loved jazz and the blues, but "Stardust" was totally unexpected. The dancing, the candles, and the music revealed his sensitive romantic side. But she knew it was that soft side of him that caused him to suffer from the things he encountered at the hospital, and she knew that side of him was being encased in a hard shell by his internship. That was fine with her as long as the shell never shut her out, and he never lost his vulnerability.

The slow dancing led to fondling, the fondling led to passionate kissing, and the kissing ended the dancing. They made love on the floor where they were dancing, they made love in one of the beanbags, and finally in the bed. They lost themselves in the physical act until they lay in each other's arms adrift on contentment.

As he held her, Dave let his mind wander, and wondered about his mass of ignited stardust. *What the hell is going on with me, with us, with our life, with all life, with death: what the hell is it all about?* All his perplexing questions could be distilled down to that one single simple question, expressed in the vernacular; what the hell is going on? He knew there was an answer to the question, but humans did not have the intellectual capacity to grasp the complexity of the question, much less the answer. Homo sapiens were not evolved enough to have the necessary intelligence to understand what the hell is going on. It would take a more advanced being, so humans had to have a philosophy of life to help them to cope with the vastness of the cosmos and their existence in it. They needed a framework to hang the fabric of their life on in order to deal with all the uncertainties and unknowns they faced daily.

For some it was religion. God determined, guided, and controlled everything. All they had to do was believe in a celestial being and have faith. For others, it was cultism. They followed a leader, a group of ideologues, or an ideology to relieve themselves of any cognitive participation. They found safety in turning themselves over to an individual, a group of individuals, or a set of rules and values.

The fabric of Dave's life was hung on mathematics, physics, biology, chemistry, and a quest for solid empirical answers. Like the ancient Greeks he admired, he used deductive reasoning to search for balance, truth, and beauty in his life. That did not mean he denied other explanations, it simply meant he only accepted what was proven. His philosophy was based on what he didn't know as much as it was based on what he did know, and he was a true agnostic, admitting there was much he did not and could not know or understand.

He had been raised Christian and he followed those teachings in his interactions with others. But he also followed the Tao, and believed he had to do the right thing, because it is the right thing to do, and to do otherwise is illogical. He read and absorbed the teachings of Siddhartha Gautama the Buddha as well as the Bhagavad Gita: so, to him life, the balance of nature, the flow of the universe, and all things in it were sacred.

Dave did not believe in organized religion. Men created organized religions, and they had all the faults, foibles, fallacies, and failings of men built into them. It never failed to amaze him how religions could twist, spin, and distort things to produce their outlandish doctrines and dogmas. He modeled his philosophy on the writings of the philosophers he read from the ancient Greeks to the Age of Enlightenment, Reason, and Humanism. He rejected existentialism and nihilism as narcissistic and self-serving excuses for negative behavior. They were forms of reasoning that legitimized despots, greedy business people, libertarians, power hungry politicians, and criminals; allowing for the exclusion of integrity and character in a society's culture. He believed education was the key to a successful society and a functional culture should be built on science and reason. *Oh well, what the hell.* He fell asleep.

The following morning Sharon slipped under his arm and put her head on his chest. "I want to keep our relationship fresh and vibrant with romantic nights like last night. I want to keep holding your stardust in my arms and dancing in our fantasy bubble." She sat up. "Don't let them take that away from us. Nothing is worth losing that part of you because that is the best part of you." They made love with the morning light filtering through the window, and it was noon before they got out of bed.

"What are we going to do today, or with what's left of today? It's your first day off in two months, and staying in the apartment is not an option, Mister Clothing Optional Man."

"I want to take a drive. I have this fantastic new car I've only driven to and from the hospital. We can find a place out in the boonies to have dinner and be back in time for some fornication."

"Are you trying to schedule our intimate time? Get it through your head, our intimate episodes happen when they happen, not on a planned schedule. Let's shower and go. I like the idea of taking a drive."

They took a bottle of chardonnay in the little cooler they used for the pool, two glasses, a blanket, and they were off: driving north on the expressway past the airport exit out into the surrounding countryside. The rural South is never far from the urban areas, so they were on a long straight stretch of freeway in the open countryside in no time. There was no traffic, so he hit a hundred and twenty, reached a hundred and thirty, then floored it, letting the car's engine wind up to its maximum high-pitched whine, before finally taking his foot off the accelerator. "God, I needed that. I feel like I left the last two months behind me somewhere on that stretch of road. Now for some real driving."

She responded. "Boys and their toys."

He took the exit onto a quintessential country lane: a curvy road that led into the forest with open fields and orchards interspersed among the trees. The children were in school, and the adults were working, so he drove as if he were driving the twenty-four hours at Le Mans. Sharon continued to sit quietly watching him as he poured all his focus into taking the curves perfectly; down shifting and accelerating again, before breaking into the next curve. She could almost see the stress related fight or flight toxins pour out of him onto the road as he intently executed each aspect of his driving. Finally, he relaxed his grip on the wheel, let his shoulders sag, and took a deep breath. "I'm alive, I'm still alive after two months of unmitigated Hell."

He began looking for a place to stop. Ahead he saw a quaint farmhouse surrounded by fields and orchards with a man at the mailbox next to the road getting his mail. Dave pulled over to talk to him. "Would you mind if we sat in your apple orchard to enjoy the afternoon? We want to put a blanket down, drink some wine, and relax. We won't disturb anything."

The man looked hard at Dave through the window, then bent down to look at Sharon smiling at him from the passenger's seat. "Sure, help yourself, just don't help yourself to any of my apples. They ain't ripe, anyway. You drive up from the city to get away from all of them people?"

Dave nodded, "You got it. Do you know of a place where we can get a bite later?"

"There is if you like German food. You go back to the freeway and head toward the city. Take the third exit on the right and drive into town. There is a German place on this side of town called The Chalet. You can't miss it because it looks like a chalet."

Sharon leaned across Dave toward the man, "Thanks, we will leave your apples alone, I promise."

"You'll enjoy the afternoon." He watched Dave drive down the gravel road that led to the gate of the orchard before returning to his house. They wandered into the orchard, spread the blanket on the grass, and he opened the wine. They were in a dense ardor of varying shades of green. The trees were filled with apples, the grass was lush, and the air was fragrant with the smell of growing things. They sat on the blanket, he poured the wine, and they clinked glasses.

She moved against him. "I want to come back here in the spring when the apple trees are in bloom and make love on this very spot surrounded by the scent of apple blossoms with their white petals raining down on us." Then her voice became soft and low as she asked, "What about next year? What kind of residency are you going to do, where do you want to do it, and what about us if you do it someplace else?"

He put his arms around her. "Whatever I do and wherever I do it, I want to be with you. I want to spend my life with you. Sharon, right here, right now, on this perfect spot, on this perfect day, I would ask you to marry me, but I know you don't want to get married, so instead I will ask you to spend your life with me. Sharon, will you spend your life with me?" She looked down and was quiet for a moment. Then the old fear and anger welled up inside her causing a knot to form in her chest. She continued to hesitate, afraid of making a commitment to him, but afraid of losing the happiness she had found with him if she didn't. Finally, she gave him an answer without any commitment. "I want to be with you, Dave."

"It would be ideal if I could do my medicine residency here. You could keep flying and things would go on just as they are for another two years. Then I want to look for a place to practice in Northern California." He pulled her down on the blanket.

"I will have five years of seniority by then. The only base we have in Northern California is San Francisco and it's a very senior base. I don't think five years is enough seniority for me to transfer there." She put her head on his chest.

"Do you want to be a flying waitress all your life? What's your degree in? You're smart enough to do anything you want." He held her close.

"When I started flying, I thought it was a glamorous profession. I love to travel, but the work is tedious and unrewarding. My degree is in Economics. I've considered going back to school part time to get my MBA while I was flying." She sat up with a look of surprise on her face. "I could get my MBA while you are doing your residency." She looked at him as if she were seeing him for the first time. "I have been worried about what was going to happen to us. I have tried to put it out of my mind and live in the moment, live in our fantasy bubble. Now I think there is a way for us to be together." She could hold on to her happiness without making a binding commitment to him, and things could go on just as they are, at least for another two years. She lay back down. "What a wonderful day, following a wonderful night."

"Let's take a walk through the orchard." They strolled through the trees, sipping wine and holding hands. They were in a shadowy green nave with the afternoon sunlight filtering through the canopy to make bright patches on the grass. They moved through the orchard from bright spot to bright spot as if they were playing a type of hopscotch in an enchanted forest where the apples looked like green Christmas ornaments hanging among the leaves. "You know we are engaged now. We are engaged to be together."

When they reached the back fence of the orchard, there was a field overgrown with wild blackberry bushes. Some of the vines protruded through the fence with big rich ripe berries dangling seductively from them. They stood at the fence, alternating between feeding each other wild blackberries, and taking sips of wine.

When the wine was finished, she left him behind as she skipped and twirled through the trees back to the blanket. He raced to catch up with her, and when he did, she pulled him down onto the blanket on top of her to kiss him. When the kiss was over, he raised himself up on his hands. "Does this mean what I think it means?"

"No, you'll have to wait until spring for what you think it means. It means I'm happy, that's all." They spent the rest of the afternoon drinking wine and talking about their future in the idyllic, peaceful setting of the orchard.

Driving back toward the farmhouse, Sharon saw the man and his wife sitting on the front porch drinking iced tea. "Stop. I want to thank him again." She got out of the car and walked to the house. "I want to thank you for letting us stop in your orchard. It's lovely and we had a wonderful afternoon."

The wife looked at her husband confused and unsure of what to say. "Would you like some iced tea?"

"No but thank you again. That orchard is very special to us now." Sharon got back in the car, and they drove off.

"I just don't understand city folks. Why would they drive all the way up here to sit in our apple orchard and think it's special? I think being all crammed up together in the city like that makes them all a little crazy." The woman shook her head.

Dave followed the man's directions to a restaurant located on the outskirts of a small dusty country town with one street. The building was an immaculately maintained perfect replica of an alpine chalet with a sign above the door that read, The Chalet. The building and beer garden looked completely out of place in the tired old town.

A pleasant, trim, blond woman dressed in an alpine costume greeted them. "I'm sorry, but we aren't open yet. You can wait in the beer garden if you'd like; the kids must finish their homework before we can open. Our daughter is the waitress, and our son is the busboy. Their schoolwork comes first. Did you drive up from the city? Are you celebrating something special?"

"Yes … we sort of … we kind of … I guess you could say … we did a type of engagement." Dave fumbled it out.

"You got engaged. That makes this an incredibly special occasion. Take this table by the window. We normally don't open until six and we are closed on Sundays. We don't work on the Lord's Day. On Sunday, we go to church and thank the Lord for our blessings. Don't worry, my husband will make a special engagement dinner for you. He is from Austria and his food is authentic Austrian cuisine. Let me suggest his specialties. His schnitzel is beyond compare, and his Tafel Spitz melts in your mouth. Let me bring you a nice fresh green salad from our garden, a wiener schnitzel, and a Tafel Spitz. You can share the main dishes. For dessert we have fresh strudel with homemade ice cream. Now, for the lady, a nice dry white wine and for the gentleman a good Austrian beer. The perfect engagement meal for such a handsome couple." She was so excited she didn't wait for an answer, or any confirmation, but rushed off to the kitchen. "Werner, we have an early guest!"

Sharon put her hands across the table to hold Dave's hands. "What a perfect way to end a perfect day."

Later a blond teenage girl in an Austrian peasant's dress appeared at their table. "I will be your waitress. Congratulations." She smiled and did a little curtsy. Behind her was a blond boy two or three years younger in lederhosen with a basket of black bread and a tub of butter. "Fresh bread and butter. Congratulations." His eyes never left Sharon as he sat the bread and butter down on the table and did a little bow. They trundled off back to the kitchen with the boy looking back over his shoulder.

"They're adorable! I feel like I am in a fairy tale. This place isn't real, and these people aren't real. We've crossed over some kind of threshold into the pages of a fairy tale. It's a magical land put here for us today." Sharon was delighted with everything that had happened since Dave entered the apartment last night.

The teenage girl brought their food, and with each course she was accompanied by the boy with a pitcher of water to refill the water glasses. The food was far beyond their expectations. When they finished, the woman appeared with six glasses of schnapps on a tray, followed by the girl, the boy, and a large man in chefs' garb. Two of the glasses had only a tiny amount of schnapps in them. She put two glasses on the table, handed the partially filled glasses to her children, took one herself, and handed the last one to the large man. "You have met my children, and this is my Werner."

Dave stood and took the large man's hand. "I am Dave, and this is Sharon. I have been to Austria, Germany, and Switzerland but this is the finest food I have ever tasted from those areas. You must be a master chef."

Werner beamed. "Thank you. Mama, you tell them why it is so good. Is not all my cooking."

"We only use home-grown ingredients from our own garden and from the farmers around here. Everything is fresh and we choose the best cuts of meat and the best produce, but he is being modest: he is a master chef. But enough about us. Sit, please, sit."

"When you drink schnapps, it is all in one drink; you finish the glass in one swallow." She held up her glass. "To you, Sharon and Dave, may you have a long life filled with love, happiness, and children to bring you joy, prost." They all repeated, "prost" and downed their glass's contents.

Sharon felt something stir inside her, a feeling she'd never felt before. She looked at the two children and an instinct she never knew she possessed rose to the surface. It was totally alien to her, but in a way, it was completely familiar. To be a mother, to have her own family, something inside her yearned for it. It was as if she had passed through a type of warp into a magical place that cast a spell over her. Mama's toast wove the spell: love, happiness, and children. If there was anything she was sure of, it was that she did not want to marry and give up her freedom, her name, and control over her life to a man. Her father, Bar, and the actor who basely raped her taught her that. And the last thing she wanted was to bring a child into the world to suffer the way she did. But now she was conflicted and confused. The little family went back to the kitchen chattering among themselves, and she sat listening to Dave lost in her own thoughts.

"I know why they are out here in the country: it's because of those two kids. They are wholesome and innocent because they aren't exposed to the negative influences of the city. They put their restaurant out here in the country for their children. They could have a top spot in the city, but they put their children first. That's the love of a mother and father."

Sharon barely heard what he said. Things she never knew existed in her were in conflict with her intellect. She sat looking at him. Maybe she did love him. He was her lover, her best friend, her companion, her soul mate, and she felt incomplete without him. She honestly thought she could never feel that way about a man. Was it simply her biological clock ticking or as Etta James sang; "at last my love has come along." Did having a mate cause feelings to formulate that give rise to natural instincts? Was it all biology, psychology, and genetic memory? Was a Darwinian creature of adaptation driven by instinct and operating on genetic memory in conflict with an intelligent thinking being. Should she listen to her heart and the very core of her being, marry Dave and have a family, or should she listen to her head and reject what she was feeling as biological instinct originating in her genetic memory, and keep things the way they are? Did she actually want to bring a child into a world filled with hate, bigotry, racism, hypocrisy, war, conflict, pain, and suffering? No, of course not. She had everything the way she wanted it. She was the happiest she had ever been, and she intended to keep it that way. Why was she overthinking such a beautiful, wonderful day. She knew why: her father.

Mama reappeared. "Please have a safe drive back to the city and may an angel rest on your bedpost tonight to bless your love." She smiled mischievously.

Sharon stood up and hugged her. "Thank you so much for the wonderful food and for a wonderful evening."

Dave thanked her and looked at her for the bill. She put her hands in the pockets of her apron and smiled. "There is no bill. Your engagement dinner is our gift to you. You remind us of ourselves, Werner, and me when we were your age, so happy and full of love. This is our way of sharing our love and happiness with you."

"We can't let you do that." Dave took out his wallet.

"You have no choice. We are blessed, and we never forget to share our blessings. I think the two of you are blessed, too. If you want to thank us, never forget to share your blessings with others." She took Sharon by the shoulders and kissed her on the cheek. "Now go, it's getting late, and we have real work to do."

"What lovely people and what a wonderful family." Dave mused as they walked to the car with their arms around each other. Sharon sat quietly in the car as they drove back to the city. She had resolved her inner conflict and was engulfed in a warm inner glow generated by their day. Dave drove the speed limit all the way back, letting the entire day soak in, and the engine hummed along the road just as quietly as its two occupants, as if it sensed their mood and was providing the proper background.

When they reached the apartment, they shed their clothes quickly, just as they shed the last two months at over a hundred and thirty miles an hour on the open road. They had solidified their relationship in an apple orchard, reinvigorated themselves with a magical dinner, and now they made love with a sense of purpose. Tomorrow, he would start a twenty-four-hour shift in the Major Medicine ER, and she would fly off on a long trip with a layover in New York City, but tonight they had each other.

When Dave walked through the automatic doors the next morning, the energy of a busy Emergency Department exploded in his face. A hospital is a living organism, and the Emergency Department is its beating heart, always pulsating with activity. He entered Major Medicine to find Henry and four fresh-faced students lounging around in the doctors' station.

Jay walked in behind him and took over. "You two are going to work with Dave, and you two are working with Henry. After you finish with your patient, present the case to your intern. He will see the patient and sign off on the chart. I know when things get rolling, we will be pressed for time, but Henry and Dave will try to do some teaching on each case. There are only two holdovers: a COPD'er finishing his treatment and an OD waiting for Psych. One last thing: you don't leave the ED. If you get a chance to sleep, you do it in one of the last exam areas in the back. We'll send a couple of you for food when it's not busy. Any questions? Good, I suggest you spend your time reading until we start getting patients."

As the students opened their Internal Medicine textbooks, Dave walked out into the hall with Henry. "Now that we have some free nights, let's get together."

"Sure, as long as we don't include Janice and Mike." Henry was seldom so emphatic about anything. He was spending more time at Sherry's and avoiding the park house as much as possible because of Mike. His issues with Mike were compounded further by Janice's constant presence. Henry's sophisticated palate simply could not accommodate Janice's perky, bubbly optimism, or her dull Kansas wit.

Jay came out into the hall to join them. "God, they look so young, but that was us only a couple of years ago. I feel so old when I look at their faces, so full of enthusiasm and zeal." Things had improved significantly for Jay since he started dressing better and taking care of his appearance. He was relaxed around Dave and Henry, his confidence had grown substantially, and he was having coffee every morning with Nurse Carol. Dave encouraged him to ask her out, but he was still too shy, and she was too professional to take things further on her own.

They needed a little encouragement and Dave felt obligated to provide that encouragement since he, Henry, and Jay had developed a close camaraderie.

The overhead came to life. "One ambulance, Code 3, for Major Medicine."

"Time to go to work, guys." Jay led them back into Major Medicine.

The overhead again, "Code 3 ambulance five minutes out."

This time from the triage desk. "Here they come."

The doors slid open, and the paramedics ran into the ER with the patient under CPR with mask, bag, and chest compressions. They stopped inside the doors and Jay checked the patient's pupils. "He is responsive." He ordered a nurse to take over the chest compressions and the code team sprang into action like the well-drilled pit crew of a race car with each member of the team performing their task quickly, efficiently, and expertly.

"Strip." Jay looked at the strip. "V-tach, stand clear." He pushed the buttons. As soon as the patient settled from the jerk of the shock, they all went back to what they were doing. "Strip." Jay looked at the second strip. "Still in V tach. Dave check his pupillary response."

Dave pulled the eyelid up and shined a light straight into the patient's eye. "Still responsive."

"Are we at three hundred jowls? What has he had IV? How many times did you shock him?" The paramedic responded and Jay put the paddles down again on the man's chest, "Good, stand clear." Jay shocked him again. "Strip. Sinus brady. Atropine one milligram."

"Atropine is in," the charge nurse replied.

"Strip. Sinus. Call the CCU and Cardiology. How about his vitals?" Jay stepped back. "Let's get him off the ambulance gurney and onto one of ours."

"His vitals are good, and his oxygen saturation is good. He is breathing on his own." The charge nurse and the ambulance crew moved the patient.

"Give me a post-resuscitation EKG." Then to the students, "Gather around and let's see what the EKG tells us. Someone call psych again, tell them the OD is cleared medically, and they need to come get her, now! Henry and Dave, once we get this guy to the CCU, one of you discharge the COPDer. What a way to start the shift."

The ambulance crew finished their paperwork and left. Psych took the OD upstairs. The resuscitated patient was transferred to the CCU, and Henry discharged the COPD'er. It was only eight o'clock and they still had another twenty-three hours to go.

"God, I haven't even had my coffee. I can't function without coffee." Henry sat down in the doctor's station.

The rest of the shift went by in typical fashion. They admitted twelve patients, treated and released another twelve, and Dave and Henry supervised the students on another dozen. They got a break in the early morning hours that allowed them to crash on the gurneys in the back: then it was over.

Henry did not leave the hospital but went to sleep in one of the call rooms in the basement, but even though he was in a stupor, Dave drove to his apartment. Sharon found him sprawled on the bed in his scrubs and OR shoes. "Dave, are you alright?"

"What time is it?" He sat up and looked around, still half asleep.

"It's after four. Was it that bad?"

"No, I just didn't want to mess up the bed." He grinned.

"Don't joke about it. You look terrible. You're in filthy scrubs and you didn't even take your shoes off." Sharon sat down on the bed.

"Don't touch me. You're right, I am covered with every type of fluid produced by the human body. I am too funky to shower in my own bathroom. Let's go to the pool and wash the big chunks off. Did you bring your bikini?" He got up.

"You haven't noticed the Sharon shelf in your closet and some unfamiliar products in your bathroom? I left a set of my essentials here with some clothes and my new bikini." She went to the closet and got their bathing suits. When he left her alone when she was undressed, she asked again. "Are you sure you're alright?"

"No, but I'll be alright, once I get the blood, piss, shit, vomit, and other stuff I don't even know what is, off me. Until I am sterilized in chlorine, I don't want you anywhere near me. But you look incredible in that new bikini, and it is only my deep affection for you and your well-being that keeps me from accosting you." Dave grinned maliciously. "Beer, I need beer, but I am afraid I will contaminate it. Can you get a beer and pour it down my throat?" She realized he was just tired, but she had never seen him look so bad, and he had lost so much weight. She went to the kitchen. "Have you eaten? Are you hungry?"

"I had breakfast yesterday and a sandwich last night. I smell too bad to eat. I need to get clean first. After I wash the big chunks off, I'll take a hot soapy soak in the tub, and we'll go out to get something. I don't want to touch the beer, just pour it down my throat." He opened his mouth and pointed to it.

"Dave, you have to eat, you're losing weight. I don't want my big strong pair bond to waste away." For months he had not eaten properly, and the lack of sleep coupled with the toll of the constant unrelenting stress was starting to show in his body. If she could see the physical effects on his body, what is it doing to him inside, psychologically, what's it doing to his emotions? She got two beers from the fridge and handed him one over his mock protest as he put his head back and pointed to his mouth for her to pour it in.

When they got to the pool, he slammed the beer down and dove in. She stood on the side of the pool watching him as he repeatedly went under water, shook out his hair, and rubbed his body. "We forgot the towels and we need more to drink. I'll go back and get the towels and more beer."

"I'm sorry Baby I had to get the ER off of me. I didn't mean to ignore you. I'll get out and get the stuff. I didn't leave the hospital at the door when I got home this morning because it was stuck all over me."

She laughed, "Don't get out; I'll get everything. I want to make sure you have the ER off of you, and the pool has time to filter it out before I get in."

She did not see him or where he came from, until he was standing in front of her. She recognized him as one of the men who followed her from the parking lot the first time she came to Dave's apartment. "Let me help you." He was nice looking, well groomed, smelled of expensive cologne, and was wearing designer board shorts. Even though he was slim and about her height, he carried the muscle bulk of someone who worked out regularly with weights. When he reached for the cooler, she smiled and said, "No thanks, I've got it."

She tried to walk around him, but he moved with her. "Where would you like to sit?"

"I'm with someone." She tried to go around him again.

The man looked over his shoulder at Dave and shrugged arrogantly. "Really, that guy? I was surprised you were with someone like him the first time I saw you. Don't you know you can do better than that? I'm Steve. Why don't you give me a chance, and I think I can convince you to trade up." He was confident and self-assured as he moved closer to her and pointed to a ground-floor apartment beside the walk. "I live right here. Let's go in, have a drink, and you know, get acquainted. He's swimming laps and neglecting you. He doesn't even know you aren't there." He put his arm around her waist and stared her toward his apartment. "What's your name? Come on in, he won't know where you are."

As soon as the man touched her, Sharon saw Dave was out of the pool in a single bound. She got a sinking feeling in the pit of her stomach when she saw the look on his face as he came striding toward them. It was the same look she saw when she told him about Bar hitting her. She pulled away from Steve, and moved quickly to put herself between him and Dave, then put her hand out in a "stop" motion. "It's okay Dave. I told him I was with someone. Now, let's go sit down."

The man turned to look, and saw Dave with his right arm partially cocked, and realized the only thing keeping him from being punched by a bigger man with the body of an athlete was the woman standing between them. Dave relaxed his right arm, but his stance did not change as he put his left arm around her and pulled her roughly to his side. He had always been so careful and gentle with her, but now his arm felt like a steel band around her. He stood with his feet planted squarely in front of the man, his left arm around her, and his right arm hanging down, but his hand was still partially in a fist. She tried to pull him away, but he was more powerful than she realized, and he held her tightly in a vice-like grip. The man smirked. "She's hot, but she's not that hot." He looked at Dave's arm and fist. "She's not worth that. But I'd keep her on a short leash, if I were you. She might wander off if you don't." She used all her strength to try to hold Dave back, but he moved easily toward the man and tightened his hand into a fist again. "That's enough." She pleaded.

That was enough for the man too, he walked away quickly, and Dave watched him with malice in his eyes as Steve scurried into his apartment and closed the door. "Dave, I deal with that kind of BS from narcissistic assholes like him all the time, and I know how to handle them. Jesus, I was so afraid you were going to hit him before I could stop you. There was no need for you to act that way. You can't just walk up to someone and punch them because you don't like the way they're talking to your girlfriend."

Dave released her and she finally relaxed. "You're right, I was going to pop him, but you got in the way; then I realized if I hit him, it would have really upset you, so I didn't. He put his hands on you, Sharon. Do you think I'm going to watch someone harass you and put their hands on you without doing anything?"

"If you're purified, let's go in. I'm not in the mood for the pool anymore." She walked back to his apartment wondering how much of that was about her and how much of it was about him being the alpha dog, the Hemingway man, the football player. That was the part of him that made her feel safe; that wild side of him that was exciting. The way he intimidated Steve without saying a word, like a big dog that didn't have to bark at a smaller yelping dog. It made her think he relished it to some degree.

Once they were in the apartment, they ended up intertwined in one of the bean bags. "I will be able to leave the hospital sometime between seven and nine tomorrow night, and I have the next day off, so we can do something. I talked to Henry about getting together. When is Labor Day? I imagine the gang will get together for a picnic, party, or something."

"Shouldn't you take it easy?" She sat up and looked at him.

He leaned back with his hands behind his head. "Stop worrying. We won't go out. We'll order in, I'll eat a whole pizza, and we can have a nice quiet evening listening to music. We've had enough excitement for one day, but I am trapped at the hospital so much of the time, I feel like I am missing most of my life. I need to get out and live every chance I get."

When he checked into Minor Medicine the next day, Dave took Henry aside. "Do you and Sherry want to meet us for dinner at one of our little neighborhood restaurants tonight?"

"Sure. I'll check with Harvin to see if he and Connie want to go too."

Minor Medicine was configured like Major Medicine only in a bigger room with more exam areas and fewer support items. Dave, Henry, Jay, and the students saw the patients as quickly as possible. The goal in Major Medicine was to get the patient stabilized, then admitted if they needed admission. In Minor Medicine, the goal was rapid turnover.

Dave waded through URIs, allergic reactions, gastroenteritis, diarrhea, asthma, rashes, headaches, anxiety attacks, depression, unwarranted fears, and drug seekers. The nonmedical psychosocial problems took up a lot of time and often created a backlog in the flow of patients.

Unlike the wards and Major Medicine where the work was difficult and stressful; in Minor Medicine it was tedious and repetitious.

The flow was steady until after lunch, when it picked up, it accelerated after five when people got off work, and peaked just before seven. Dave called Sharon and told her they were going to dinner at the Italian place. The three of them, along with the students, worked through dinner and finished a little after seven.

The restaurant was decorated with old-world charm and had a distinct Lady and the Tramp feel to it. Like the Mexican restaurant, it was family owned and operated, with the mama doing the cooking using her family recipes to produce home-style comfort food. Once the greetings were over and they were all seated, Harvin informed them, "Connie and I have set a date and I'm applying for a straight Medicine internship in California at UCSF, Stanford, USC, and UCLA. With her credentials Connie can get a job at the hospital where I'm doing my internship. I graduate in May and we're getting married the first week in June. My parents are paying for a big wedding and a two-week honeymoon in Saint- Tropez."

When the waiter arrived, Henry ordered three bottles of Chianti. Once the wine was opened and poured, they clinked glasses, and toasted Harvin and Connie. Dave added, "I'm applying for a Medicine residency at those same places and here. Sharon is going back to school to get her MBA while I'm doing my residency. She's applying to the graduate business schools at UC Berkeley, Stanford, UCLA, USC and of course here."

Sherry's eyes widened. "Are you sure you can get into those MBA programs in California, Sharon?"

"I did get two Bs in college, but they were in PE and an elective, not my major. I majored in economics. I got a B in an elective because the TA hit on me and I turned him down, so he made sure I didn't get an A. I got a B in PE because I refused to do some dumb stuff, they made us do."

Sherry could not control her reaction. "You're tall and you're beautiful! That should be enough. But you're smart too?" Sherry was jealous of Sharon's looks and height, but her solace had always been that she had an MBA from Duke.

The waiter reappeared, but Henry told him to wait until they called him, then asked Dave and Harvin why they were applying in California. Dave replied, "I plan to stay there permanently. The ocean and mountains are only a couple of hours apart for sailing and skiing. San Francisco and LA are great cities with everything you could want and there's hope for the future out there, you can feel it in the air, it's almost electric. Here all you feel is the toxicity of the past."

Henry pressed the point. "What about you, Sharon, and Connie? Are you on board with this or are you just following your men?"

Sharon answered, "I would prefer to stay here, but I wouldn't mind getting out of the South. I'm tired of the misogyny and sexual harassment. I couldn't walk to the pool yesterday without a guy blocking my way and trying to pull me into his apartment. I've had layovers in both LA and San Francisco. I can think of a lot worse places, and to tell you the truth, fewer better places to live."

Connie followed with, "Harvin and I have discussed where we want to live. With Harvin's family's support we can go anywhere we want, and we decided on California for the same reasons; the weather, the beaches, the mountains: you name it, like Dave said, California has it all." Connie looked at Sharon. "I get the harassment thing, too. I deal with it a lot at the hospital."

They looked at their menus in silence until Henry called the waiter over. After they ordered Connie brought it up, "What about you, Henry? What are your plans? What are you going to do?"

"Until now, it's been a matter of course: get my degree and get a good internship, but I never thought past that. Because of my financial position, I have advantages far beyond most people, and I feel I should use those advantages to do something significant. I know it sounds like a cliché, but I believe in noblesse oblige. I think humanity will face more epidemics and pandemics in the future. I want to help deal with those upcoming catastrophes. I'm going to do an infectious disease fellowship, hopefully at Hopkins, and try to do pure research at the CDC. I think the front line of our defense against the plagues that are coming will be there, and I want to make a contribution to the fight." Henry looked at Sherry. "I'm sorry I didn't tell you sooner."

Henry could live for himself, like his cousins and sister, but instead he chose a life of purpose. He was a world-class swimmer who could have won Olympic medals, but he gave that up to pursue his education and go to medical school. He could be a Park Avenue internist, mingle with the rich and powerful; celebrities, actors, politicians, and business leaders, but instead he was going to confine himself to a lab to prevent thousands, if not millions of deaths. Henry was called.

Sherry was overwhelmed and confused. How could she be disappointed that she wasn't going to be a New York socialite because Henry was going to be saving humanity? She felt betrayed, yet knowing what Henry wanted to do made it hard for her to justify her feelings. She wasn't a bad person, but she was a product of her class, raised in wealth and privilege. She was smart, educated, and aware; that side of her saw Henry as noble, but her other side was spoiled and self-focused, so she remained silent.

After dinner, Dave offered, "Why don't we go back to our place and listen to some music?" Sharon had moved more of her stuff into Dave's apartment and the only time she spent at her house was when he was at the hospital. She liked the sound of it, "our place."

Henry looked at Sherry. "I think we better pass."

At his apartment, the girls talked about Henry and Sherry until Dave interrupted. "Henry is using Sherry and Sherry wants to use Henry. Sherry is like every girl Henry dated in college: pretty, wealthy, refined, sophisticated, and selfish. Henry needs a woman to take care of him and he needs them to be cut from that same cloth. He's never been serious about a girl. If Sherry dumps him, he will find another one just like her. That's what he did in college. Henry doesn't believe in love; he is too pragmatic and unemotional. He protects himself from any drama or physiological entanglements. He's my best friend and I love him like a brother, but I know him. When he's ready he'll look for a permanent mate, his term, not mine, and when he does, he'll base his selection on a whole host of criteria, not love."

"Do you really believe that?" Sharon liked Henry and she was surprised by what Dave said.

Dave continued. "I don't just believe it, I know it. Believe me, I know Henry and he knows me. How accurate was he when he told you about me?"

"He was very accurate; except he didn't tell me what an asshole you can be sometimes." Sharon did not like what Dave said about Henry.

Connie sat up. "I think that's a given. The asshole part, I mean. If he is a man, he is an asshole to some degree. It is only a matter of degrees. We women know we must put up with some degree of assholishness, but if the asshole is cute and the assholishness is manageable, we're okay with it, we women are very tolerant."

"You men are lucky we women put up with as much as we do. We even take you inside our bodies to satisfy your desires, but we will only accept a certain amount of assholishness. If your assholishness becomes unmanageable, we will find another asshole to lavish our womanliness on." Sharon sat up and looked at Dave.

"What did I do this time to be called an asshole this time?" Dave asked.

"You are man, that's what you did. But you are a cute, manageable asshole, so I guess I will keep letting you inside my body." Sharon settled back in Dave's arms.

Harvin pulled Connie back down. "How about me?"

"Well, I have been letting you inside my body for over a year, and I am going to marry you, so I guess you are good to go." She laughed. "It would be so much fun if we were together in California."

Harvin added, "Except for a couple of things like residency and internship. But we won't let trivial things like that get in our way and spoil our fun, will we?" Connie and Harvin stayed at Dave's apartment talking, listening to music, and drinking wine until after midnight.

Sharon woke up the next morning, found her clothes, pulled a pair of shorts out of his closet, and threw them at him. "Let's get out of this apartment." He got up but would not leave her alone while she was dressing. "Am I going to have a problem with you?" She stopped him and pushed him away, but he came right back for her. "Is there something wrong with us? We are at each other every chance we get. Is that normal?"

"It's normal as far as I can see." He would not be deterred and guided her to the bed.

Afterwards, as they lay in bed, Dave said, "I don't think there is something wrong with us. I think there is something right with us."

She snuggled against him. "Dave are we always going to be this happy? I hope so. I love our life and our friends. I love things the way they are now." They got out of bed, showered, dressed, and drove to her house.

On the way, they bought a bottle of Pinot Noir, a baguette, two types of cheese, a salami, an apple, a pear, and some chocolates. They walked to a nice spot in the park and set up their picnic like two children off on a lark on a balmy late summer day. The sky was a cloudless bright blue, the grass was a deep, rich green, the air temperature was pleasant and pleasing.

"When your lease is up, we can move in together. I want two bedrooms. One will be our bedroom: the other will be our study. It has to have a kitchen, but I don't intend to use it. I've never learned to cook, and I don't intend to learn now. I want an inviting, sophisticated look that reflects our personalities."

Her eyes were bright, and her face seemed to glow as she gazed off in the distance, picturing her first home with Dave. Saying "our place" had triggered something domestic in her. Making plans for her home with him was more pleasant than she thought it would be. "I know we have to move into an apartment because you will want a pool. You're such a water guy, but no singles apartment. I have to put up with unwanted attention at work, but I am not going to put up with it where I live." She looked dreamy again. "I want to live with you. I want us to spend the evenings reading, talking, listening to music, and our nights making love in our own bed, in our own home."

She looked up to see Bob and Phil standing over them with a bottle of wine and a blanket. "We saw you and thought we would join you." Phil spread their blanket, and they sat down. "Are you going to make it to our Labor Day Happening? We're having the gang over for wine and cheese. Everyone has to work the next day, so we won't go late."

"I'll be coming off a twenty-four-hour shift in the ER and I won't even be up until late afternoon."

Bob pleaded, "Come anyway. Gorgeous, we never see you anymore. Halloween is coming up and that is the biggest party night on the park. We're going to throw the wildest, most outrageous Halloween party the Park has ever seen. You have to make that."

They spent the afternoon with Bob and Phil lounging in the warm sunshine talking and drinking wine. When they returned to the apartment, they were mellow and refreshed, and Sharon grew pensive sitting in a bean bag with him. "I am not going to be the hot young flight attendant and you are not going to be the handsome dedicated young intern forever. This time of our life is precious. We need to savor and enjoy every minute of it, because when it's over, it will be gone forever. I know you're going through a tough time at the hospital, but I love our life here with all our friends. I know you want to go to California, but I want to stay here, and I want things to go on the way they are. I really hope you get accepted here." She was happy, and happiness had been hard for her to find. Now that she had found it, she didn't want to take a chance of losing it. Talking about going to California next year had shaken her happiness and caused it to wobble a little. She didn't sleep well that night.

Dave liked the smell of the ED. It was a sharp, clean, antiseptic odor that produced an immediate psychological response like the smell of a locker room in a stadium before a game. When he arrived in the Major Medicine ER the Sunday morning of Labor Day weekend, that smell launched him into total chaos. There wasn't enough room in the Minor Medicine waiting area and the patients were spilling out onto the sidewalk. The triage area was swamped, all the exam areas in Minor and Major Medicine were occupied and there were patients on gurneys in the main hall. The senior resident, the junior residents, the interns, and students from the previous shift were still seeing patients in Major and Minor Medicine. With all four teams working, they cleared the patients from the hall and freed up a couple of exam areas by ten o'clock

The uncontrollable, bizarre acting drunks; the GI bleeds and intractable vomiting caused by alcohol or drugs; the psych cases and delusional states; and the drugged or drunk unconscious patients; all mixed with patients with pulmonary issues, cardiac problems, diabetes, and a whole plethora of other medical problems to produce an unmanageable toxic mixture of smells, noises, and visual horrors. The ambulance bay was full, with ambulances coming and going for the entire twenty-four hours; hauling the broken, battered, shattered, convulsing tide of humanity in extremis to the overwhelmed, overworked, over stressed doctors, students, and nurses who were physically exhausted and emotionally drained by the end of their shifts.

Things occurred during Dave's internship that he was never able to talk about or think about. He repressed them because they were too painful or affected him too deeply. Other things occurred he could never forget; they were always as vivid in his mind as if they had just happened. One of those things occurred later that morning.

He was running a code on a patient who had arrived by ambulance, Henry was trying to control a patient with multiple seizures in in the hall, Jay was lavaging and pushing blood on a GI bleeder as he bled out in an exam area, the senior resident was dealing with an OD, and all four students were over their heads with patients beyond their capabilities.

A biker was brought in by his gang unconscious from drugs and alcohol. His blood alcohol was off the chart and his toxicology would take some time, so Jay told a nurse to start a large bore IV on him, push fluids, put a Foley catheter in him, and give him Narcan. Then the biker was put in an exam area in the back of the ER and forgotten.

Dave had finished putting a chest tube in a patient with a pneumothorax in the last exam area at the back of the ER, when he heard the crash of a Mayo stand going over, and the sound of shattering glass. One of the nurses rushed toward the exam area where the sounds came from as the biker emerged with a broken bottle in one hand and his Foley catheter in the other.

"Get this out of my cock!" He screamed as he waved a broken bottle like a broken beer bottle in a bar fight. He backed the nurse off until she was behind Dave, and they were both trapped at the back of the ER with the biker blocking their way. "I'm going to cut you for sticking this tube in my dick!" He advanced on them with the broken bottle at the ready.

Dave was standing beside a Mayo stand with an open chest tube packet on it. He grabbed the chest trocar in his right hand and jerked the Mayo tray off the stand to hold as a shield in his left hand. "I'm a doctor and I know exactly where your heart is. It's right there at your fourth rib." He thrust the trocar at the biker's chest. "You may cut me, but this is designed to penetrate the chest wall. I'll drive it into your heart, and you will be dead by the time you hit the floor."

The biker realized the trocar was a much better weapon than a broken bottle, plus Dave looked capable of doing exactly what he said. He lowered the broken bottle and waved the foley catheter tube at Dave. "I am getting out of here. I want this out of my cock." He was focused on the trocar leveled at his chest, so he didn't see or hear the two security guards come through the doors. The night stick made the sound of a ripe melon breaking open on the back of his head, and he went down with the two guards on him immediately. One put his knee in the middle of the biker's back and held up his hands for the other to zip tie. Then they rolled him over, zip tied his feet together, jerked him up, and slammed him down on the gurney in the exam area he came from. They had him in four-point restraints in no time. Dave heard another sound like a cleaver hitting meat, then the two security guards emerged.

"You alright, Doc?" He was still holding the trocar in his shaking hand, but the shaking in his hand was nothing compared to the quivering going on inside him. His whole core felt like a bowl of jelly slopping around. "If you mean, am I hurt, no he didn't hurt me. If you mean, am I alright, hell no, but thanks, guys. I don't know what would have happened if you hadn't gotten here when you did."

"We saw you stand him down as we came through the doors. We just put him down. You had him under control. He is going to need stitches in his head and his nose isn't where it is supposed to be. He must have hit his face on the floor when we took him down." They looked at each other with the faint hint of a smile. "We'll notify the city police, and they will pick him up when you're through with him."

Dave put the trocar down and put his hand out. "Thanks again."

They both shook his hand. "Don't worry Doc, we've got your back. We'll never let anything happen to any of our people if we can prevent it, but you're the one who kept him from hurting someone. I know you were scared, but give yourself some of the credit, you're the one who protected your staff. What you did took guts."

"It wasn't like I had a choice. I was the staff who was going to get hurt." The two guards smiled. Everyone was standing around listening. All the other doctors, nurses, and students said something to him, patted him on the back, or touched him in some way. "I need to sit down for a minute. Give me a minute to get it together before I pick up the next patient." He went to the doctor's station and sat down.

Dave left the ER on Monday morning around ten, got to his apartment, fell on the bed, and was asleep in no time. He woke up at four and stumbled into the front room to find Sharon in one of the beanbags reading his psychiatry textbook. "Dave, you look terrible. I am afraid the ER is going to kill you."

"It almost did." He mumbled.

"What?"

"Nothing, let me get ready and we'll go."

Phil greeted them when they arrived. "Gorgeous, there is wine and cheese on the small table. Help yourself then come sit with me. Dave, you find your own place to sit. You have had her," Phil paused and smiled at Sharon, "and now you have to share." Phil patted a place beside him on the couch.

Dave poured them two glasses of wine, Sharon sat down beside Phil, and Dave sat on the floor beside Mike. Caroline waited until everyone was settled then said, "Now that we are all here, I have an announcement. Ron and I are getting married in April." She held out her hand to show them a large solitaire diamond on her ring finger.

Phil offered a toast. "To two of the nicest people I know, congratulations."

Bob added to Phil's toast. "Wow, first Connie and Harvin, now Caroline and Ron, and I think others are going to follow. Best wishes to you all."

The women clustered around Caroline to look at the ring and hug her. After the excitement over Caroline and Ron settled down, Dave told them, "Sharon and I are moving in together as soon as my lease is up."

Phil offered another round of toasts. "To those engaged, those about to be engaged," he leered at Sharon, "and those planning to live in sin, congratulations to you all."

Mike did not drink that toast or say anything, but his dark, cloudy brow spoke volumes. Dave did not notice, but Sharon did. His look sent a frigid chill through her, and she realized Mike might be more than creepy: he might be dangerous. Sharon had dismissed his late-night visit from her mind, but now she wondered if she should have been more forceful in her rejection of him. Could she have created a problem by leaving the door open for him, even though it was only open a crack? She was unaware that the festering seed she had planted that night had sprouted into a poisonous plant that was continuing to grow.

The rest of the month in the Medicine ED ground on with no respite just as the first two months on the Medicine wards had. Twenty-four hours in the Major Medicine ER every fourth day was taking more of a toll on Dave than every third night on call on the Medicine wards had. After breakfast, he was lucky to get a sandwich during the whole shift, then he went home the next day and fell asleep immediately. Not eating, along with the stress and lack of sleep, were causing him to lose more weight. He had an athlete's body: trim and balanced, with broad shoulders, well defined arms and legs, and a deep chest. He had always been proud of his body, but now it was melting away.

When he was not at the hospital, Sharon tried to make sure he ate, and she enticed him to bed, so he got enough sleep, but nothing she did seemed to help. The weight kept dropping off him with each passing week. The thing that worried her most was what the stress was doing to him inside. What unseen and undetected damage was he suffering?

He was sitting in Major Medicine one evening feeling down because he had run two codes and neither had been successful. When a patient was down for a long time, he could cope with losing them. But if CPR had been started quickly and there was a chance of reviving them, he had a tough time coping with a failed resuscitation. Knowing he was the one who gave up, and called the code always made him feel like he was the patient's judge, jury, and executioner. The worst part was having to tell the family he was unable to save their loved one.

A small mixed-race man arrived in four-point restraints on a gurney with straps across his knees, his waist, and his chest. There were two large city police officers at the foot of the gurney and two big burly firefighters, instead of paramedics, at the head of the gurney.

Jay looked at the extreme measures taken to immobilize the man and said, "We'll take it from here. You can take the restraints off."

One of the firefighters responded. "I don't think you want to do that, Doc."

"Of course, I do. He's unconscious. How can I examine him tied down like this?"

The firefighter tried to tell him the man had trashed the inside of the ambulance, injured a paramedic, and that it took all four of them to get him restrained in the first place: but Jay cut him off. "I said take the restraints off. This man is unconscious, and I need to examine him immediately."

The firefighter was still concerned. "Do you take full responsibility for him if we untie him?"

"I am the resident in charge here, of course I take full responsibility." Jay bristled. "This man needs attention. Now, take the restraints off."

The man waited until the last restraint was off, opened his eyes, then went after the two police officers at the end of the gurney, tipping it up and over as he went off the end. He took the police officers down, kicking and punching them. The two firefighters looked at each other, then jumped into the fray. A Code Gray was called, and two big security guards responded to join the fight. They all crashed into the supply shelves on the wall, bringing them down to the sound of breaking glass. It looked like a cartoon with one of the men flying out of the pile backwards from time to time, only to get up, and jump back in. At one point, the little man was up and all six of the men, who were twice his size, were down. They finally subdued him.

All six of the men were bruised and bloody, but the little man was relatively unscathed. The big firefighter who had spoken before had an innocent look on his face as he said, "Do you want us to untie him again Doc or did you get all your examining done that time?" Even though everyone in the ER was horrified, they could not help laughing.

Dave rotated off the Medicine service in survival mode. He left the Minor Medicine ER on his last day, drove to his apartment, and dressed for dinner with Sharon at an expensive French restaurant in the park Area to celebrate.

Helen answered the door when he got to the house. "I know, you're here for Sharon, but I didn't know you were here to take her away."

Sharon came down the stairs in a green cocktail dress that matched the green in her eyes, a darker green wrap draped over her shoulders, and matching heels. "Where are you guys going?" Helen was waiting at the door with Dave.

"To Paris," Sharon said, as she swept out the door. She took Dave's arm as they walked along. "I wish we were in Paris tonight. We would have drinks at the hotel, dinner at a romantic café, then go to a jazz club on the Left Bank."

"I promise you that night in Paris someday." He looked at her in the low light of the streetlamps and felt something stir deep inside him that was so intense it was almost painful. What he felt was not motivated by her beauty or his passion for her physically; it was a gut-wrenching emotion emanating from the very center of his being caused by his overwhelming love for her; for her goodness, her kindness, and her gentleness. He wanted to protect her and shield her from the harshness of the world. She was too soft for the hard cruelty he knew was out there.

They walked on to the restaurant pretending they were walking to a cafe in Paris. It was a perfect early autumn night and they felt like they had the world all to themselves as they walked silently along the sidewalk in the soft glow of the streetlights. They did not want to break the spell of the evening by talking, so they walked quietly along holding hands.

The restaurant was not crowded, and they were seated at a nice table by a window overlooking the lake in the park. "I know you are worried about me but I'm okay. I've lost some weight, and I have a few dings, but I am intact. I don't feel the same about a lot of things, but I am still me. I'm going to get through this; we're going to get through this. I'm going to be fine; we're going to be fine. There's only one more hard rotation, not that the other two are easy, but the OB/GYN and Pedi rotations are nothing like Medicine and Surgery. I can do this; we can do this. There are some things I will never forget and there are some things I have to forget. I have to repress them and deny them, so I suppress them deep inside me in a place I never go. That may not be healthy, but I have learned how to do it. I've been through the fire, and I may be scorched, but I'm not burned. I've grown up and matured, that's all. Surgery is going to be tough, and I may come out of that rotation battered and bruised, but I'll still be me. After my Medicine rotation, I know that now. Remember Invictus by Henley, 'my head is bloody but unbowed.' I may come out of internship bloody, but I will be unbowed. I'll still be me, maybe a leaner, more mature, grown-up version of me, but still me." He raised his glass to her. "One down and three to go, and I, we're, halfway through the worst of it." They clinked glasses. It was a learning curve, and like all learning curves, it had taken time for him to master it.

Chapter 5

The Surgery Wards

The Surgery chief resident was waiting for him when he reported to the nurse's station on the surgery floor. He gave Dave a quick orientation and introduced him to his team. The orientation was short, and the introductions were clipped, because his team had to get back to their morning rounds and elective surgeries.

Surgery teams at University Hospital are made up of one student, one intern, one junior resident (first or second year), and one senior resident (third or fourth year), and like the Medicine teams, they stayed together for a three-month rotation. They were on call every third day and made rounds every morning. They did elective surgeries in the morning and clinic in the afternoon on the day before call and follow-up rounds the morning after call, but no clinic so they could leave the hospital after rounds.

Unlike the two students Dave worked with for a month in the Medicine ED, he would be with this student for three months. His name was Jason, and he was a typical kiss ass gunner only concerned about his grades and rank in class. The junior resident was Richard, a second-year resident from a good school who did his internship at University Hospital. He was calm, steady, and quiet with a decidedly conservative outlook. The senior resident was Tom, a third-year resident who attended an Ivy League medical school and was the exact opposite of Richard. He was big, loud, brash, and cocky with a personality that overshadowed everyone around him. His hair was short, like his temper, but he was long on intolerance, and more conservative than Richard.

Richard and Tom had been together for three months and they got along amazingly well because Richard never said anything, and

Tom never shut up. They immediately decided Dave was a rotator who would not make a contribution to the team, and they dealt with him by ignoring him. He would have to change their attitude toward him by proving himself, and he knew the best way to accomplish that was to do his job.

Tom told him they did everything together. "We made rounds at seven and we operate in pairs. You'll operate with Richard, and Jason will operate with me, but he goes to class in the afternoon during the week. We eat breakfast, lunch, and dinner together, and we hang out together in the doctor's lounge. We leave the hospital at the same time and walk out together. We're finished after Grand Rounds on Saturdays if we're not on call, and usually by ten on Sundays if that's not a call day."

They did not meet with an attending, and there were no rounds with the chief. The only time he saw the chief of Surgery was at Grand Rounds on Saturday, and the attending only operated with the residents on the most difficult cases. Their team was on call the next day, so he left the hospital after clinic. Sharon was on a layover, so he spent the night alone wondering how to deal with the difficult personalities of his team members.

The next day they finished their rounds and were in the lounge when the ER resident called Tom with an admission. They smelled the patient before they saw him. The ER resident handed each of them a mask and put one on himself. When he opened the curtain of the exam area, the smell was so overpowering, it turned their stomachs, and Jason started gagging.

"I've seen some gross things, but this is as gross as it gets." The resident pulled the sheet back from the leg of a small Latino man in his sixties and the smell completely overwhelmed them. Jason threw up in his mask and started to collapse.

Dave caught him and called for ammonia capsules. He popped an ammonia capsule and stuck it in front of Jason's mask, but as soon as he started to revive, he saw the man's leg, and went down again. Dave laid him on the ER floor, turned him over to a nurse, and stuck the remaining ammonia capsules in his pocket.

The smell was bad, but the sight of the man's leg was worse. His lower leg was rotten, with maggots squirming in the putrid flesh. They were wiggling and crawling in his leg, on his foot, and between his toes. The man was a diabetic with peripheral vascular disease, and he had lost the blood supply to his lower leg causing it to necrose. The maggots probably saved his life by eating away the dead flesh. The ER resident told them, "His family has been afraid to bring him in because he's illegal, so they let his leg rot until they couldn't stand the smell anymore. This is a simple amputation to remove a dead leg, so I didn't call Ortho. I thought you guys could handle it. We typed and crossed him for four units, cultured his leg and blood, drew all his labs, and started a big bore IV with normal saline. He is all yours. Oh, don't try to kill the smell with air freshener; it only makes it worse."

"Call the OR and tell them to get ready for an AK amputation and to notify anesthesia. Richard, you and Dave take this one. Jason is worthless." Richard knew Tom was using Jason as an excuse to get out of an unpleasant task, but he had learned the way to get along with Tom was to never question anything he did or said, so he went to the doctor's station to write an admit note and pre-op orders.

Dave swallowed hard to calm his quivering stomach, tried not to vomit, and dove in. "I want a gallon of saline, two suture sets, some plastic bags, a big bowl, a gallon of betadine, and a nurse who can handle herself. Also, see if one of the nurses has any perfume with them; if they do, put some on two masks."

In no time the charge nurse showed up with everything and laid it all out in the exam area. "I can't ask one of my girls to do this." The charge nurse handed him one of the perfumed masks, put the other one on, and situated the big bowl under the man's leg.

Dave opened a suture set, took the tweezers, and scissors out, and handed the other set to the charge nurse. He poured saline over the leg, wiped the dead tissue and maggots off, used tweezers to pick out the embedded ones, and the suture scissors to cut away the dead flesh. It took them about an hour to debride the leg because they had to stop from time to time to get away from the smell and quell their nausea. When they finished, he poured betadine over the leg, put it in a plastic bag, and taped the bag to the man's thigh. The nurse dumped the contents of the big bowl into another plastic bag and tied it shut.

"Someone take this out and dump it in the proper place." He took his masks off, because the smell was finally clearing, thanked the charge nurse, and walked back to the doctor's station. "He is ready when the OR is ready for us. He needs a Medicine consult. I'll call them." Richard didn't say anything, but Dave could tell his first impression of him had changed.

The amputation went smoothly with Dave demonstrating he could suture, cut, tie, and use both hands with dexterity, so by the end of the case, he was doing his side and Richard was doing the other side. Richard looked at him, their eyes met, and from the look of respect he got, Dave knew he had proven himself.

"Go ahead and close. I'll dedicate the op note." Richard left him to close the stump with the scrub nurse. *One down and one to go.* It took him a while to close because they had taken the leg extremely high to get viable tissue, so the stump wound was large, and it required a drain. All of that took time, so when he got back to the lounge, Tom greeted him with a snide comment about how long he took. Dave ignored him. He would be working with Richard, and he had established himself with him, so Tom was superfluous, but he could not ignore Jason. He chimed in an attempt to ingratiate himself with Tom. Dave was a doctor and Jason was a student. He couldn't allow a student to insult him.

"You know you're going to hurt yourself fainting every time you see a few maggots eating some guy's rotten leg." Dave still had the ammonia capsules from the ER in his pocket. He walked over to where Jason was sitting, put them in the breast pocket of his scrubs, and smashed them all with his open hand. The excessive ammonia smell hit Jason in the face like a brick, and that coupled with the memory of the maggots, drove him to the bathroom vomiting.

Tom laughed out loud. "That was great!" *So, all I have to do to keep you off my back is be a bully, like you?* He understood that tormenting Jason had made him one of them in Tom's eyes: a tough, take no prisoners, hard-ass surgeon. The rest of Dave's shift went by smoothly. He and Richard did an appendectomy, Tom and Jason did a small bowel resection for obstruction due to adhesions and a hot gallbladder. The team also did several consults. Dave was able to rest during the day sprawled out on a couch in the doctor's lounge, and sleep that night in one of the surgery call rooms.

He had learned how to sleep in any position, any place, any time as a student. He could sleep sitting up, standing up if he had something to lean against, and one time had fallen asleep holding a retractor in surgery. No one knew he was asleep, even when he woke up with a start, and moved the retractor. The only comment came from the resident telling him to hold the retractor still.

The next morning, they were out of the hospital by noon. Sharon returned from her trip in the early afternoon and found him sitting in a beanbag; listening to music; drinking a beer. "Connie called about the Halloween party. She said everyone is getting together tonight at the park house to plan it. We can have an early dinner then drop by for a while. The day before Halloween is my last day on call on the Surgery wards, so I should get out of the hospital around noon on Halloween. My first day in the Surgery ER is an off day, so we're good to go for the party." He went to the fridge for another beer and poured Sharon a glass of wine. "I've been thinking, you need to look into the MBA programs here and in California if you're going to do that while I'm doing in residency."

She joined him in a beanbag. "So, we actually could be going to California next year?" She slid under his arm and put her head on his chest. The smell of her Chanel and the touch of her body acted like a drug on him. He pulled her to him, kissed her, and let his hands roam over her trim figure, losing himself in her the way he always did. "We don't have time for that. You'll have to wait. Do you really think things are different in California: is it better out there, or is that just a dream, a California dream?"

He sat up. "Most of humanity doesn't want anything better. If you try to fix what is wrong with humanity, they will kill you for your effort: Socrates, Buddha, Jesus, Gandhi, Dr. King. I like the line from Symphony for the Devil: 'they shouted out, who killed the Kennedys, when after all, it was you and me.'"

She sat up beside him. "I think you're right. Take all the carnage caused by religion. More people have been killed, tortured, and maimed in the name of God than anything else in history. Your God, my God, the best God, the right God, you name it. Look at the history of Christianity. The Pope duped poor people into giving money to build a huge cathedral, and when Martin Luther spoke out against what he was doing, it triggered the reformation, which led to the Hundred Years War. A war among Christians over the same God that lasted a hundred years and is still causing trouble. Tell me how the Sermon on the Mount or the Beatitudes justified the Spanish Inquisition. The greed of Christian knights caused the crusades, a war between Christianity and Islam that is still going on today. And don't get me started on Islam, that peaceful religion that was spread by jihad, 'Convert or die. There can only be peace in the world when the entire world is Muslim.' Not to mention how it treats women. They still kill each other over who should have succeeded Mohamed. How many people died as that peaceful religion was spread throughout Africa, the Middle East, India, the Caucuses, and Europe? And don't forget the Jews and their never-ending wars with the Arabs. I almost forgot the witch burnings. How many tens of thousands of women were burned to death because of religion?"

Dave responded, "Hope is the only thing humans have in this world. That's what sustains us in the face of everything else. Camus was right, life is absurd, but we can give it meaning through love, and love generates hope." They were silent for some time, lost in their own thoughts, but they felt secure in the fact they had each other even though all the turmoil of the outside world was swirling around them.

Everyone was at the park house when they arrived. Phil started by telling them how important it was to keep things from getting out of control because of the police presence around the park on Halloween night. Sherry went over what they were going to provide and how they were going to pay for it. "We are going to have beer and wine in the dining room with a bowel for people to put money in." Harvin talked about the music. "A guy in our class worked part time as a DJ in college doing weddings. He is going to provide the music for weed, wine, and beer, for him and his date. We will push all the chairs and couches in both rooms against the walls to make room to dance." Bob explained about the costume contests. "We're going to give gift certificates from our store as prizes for the best costumes. The categories are Best Costume, a hundred dollars; Sexiest Costume, a hundred dollars: Best Couples Costumes, two hundred dollars. If you go for the sexiest costume, my advice is to show more skin than costume. We will vote on the categories to get the party started. Also, anyone who wants to decorate can do it the day before the party."

Phil added that the cops would shut everything down after midnight so everyone should plan to sleep in one of the three houses on the park. "We know everyone who lives in the park area will be going from party to party, but Halloween on the Park is an adult affair, so we won't get any trick-or-treaters. No sane parent would let their child trick-or-treat around the park." They drove back to his apartment after spending time with their friends. Tomorrow he would be back with Jason, Richard, and Tom, but tonight he was with her, and the hospital was forgotten in her arms.

He found the Surgery wards less taxing than the Medicine wards. There was more down time when he was at the hospital, a half-day off after call, and a lot less stress because the senior resident made all the decisions and took all the responsibility. He was able to eat breakfast, lunch, and dinner every day, so his weight stabilized. The only downside was fatigue from standing in the OR for long hours.

Jason couldn't forget or forgive the humiliation of the ammonia capsule incident, and that was causing friction between them, so Dave decided to try to defuse the situation. They were called to the ER for a patient with appendicitis. He had done several appendectomies with Richard assisting him, so Dave asked Tom to let him take this one with Jason. Tom looked at Richard, who nodded, so he shrugged and said, "Sure."

All Jason had done up until then was hold a retractor for Tom, but Dave let him tie and cut under close supervision, making him do it over until it was perfect. Then he let Jason close. He was patient and helpful, teaching Jason how to do things right, without being harsh or critical. Tom greeted them with one of his usual cryptic comments when they got back. "How many appendices did that guy have? He must have had at least three as long as you two took."

"It took a while because I let Jason tie, cut, and close. He did fine. I think he can make a real contribution to the team now." Dave responded, and Jason walked confidently to a couch without saying a word with a look of pride on his face.

It took a patient coding in post-op, and an incident with Sharon for Tom to finally fully accept him. He got to the patient first, ran the code, and the patient survived. Tom didn't like Dave's liberal attitude, but he respected his work ethic, his knowledge, and his ability to use his hands. He began to ignore his attitude after the code.

The incident with Sharon occurred because Dave's car needed service. He was on call in the middle of the week, Sharon had a turn-around, and they were both off the next day. So, they got up early, she followed him to the dealership where he did a key drop for the service, and took him to the hospital before driving to the airport.

The next day she picked him up at the entrance to the staff parking lot. The team walked out together as usual, and they were walking toward the parking lot when Tom saw her standing beside her car. She was dressed in tight skinny jeans, ankle boots with heels, and a fuzzy red sweater with an oversized neck that dropped off one shoulder with the sleeves pushed up to her elbows.

Tom reacted immediately, "Jesus, look at that babe. Watch the big dog work and no little dog better get between the big dog and his bone." He walked straight up to her with the others trailing behind him.

She smiled at Dave and asked, "How was your night?"

"It wasn't bad, Baby." Dave walked past Tom, put his arm around her, and kissed her.

Tom blurted out. "You're Baby!"

"Sharon, this is my surgery team, Tom, Richard, and Jason. Guys, this is Sharon Kelly."

She turned on a huge smile and her eyes lit up as she stepped toward Tom, putting her hand out. He looked at her in disbelief, took her hand, and was actually speechless for once. Then she offered her hand to Richard and Jason in turn, smiling and saying how pleased she was to meet them.

"Let's get going." Dave walked around to get in the passenger's side of the car.

Richard, who never said anything, was the only one who spoke. "I hear Dave on the phone with you at night. It is nice to meet you and finally know who he is talking to."

She beamed at him, told him it was her pleasure, tossed her hair, got in the car, and waved to them as she drove away.

Jason exclaimed. "Who would have thought Baby looked like that!"

But it was Tom who echoed what they were all thinking, "I wonder who she is and what someone that hot is doing with Dave?"

The next morning, Tom pounced on him immediately. "Who is she?"

Dave was nonchalant and acted coy. "Who is who?"

"What do you mean, who's who? You know what I mean. The hot babe who met you at the parking lot yesterday?" Tom didn't like being played.

"She's Sharon Kelly, I introduced you, remember." Dave pretended to be disinterested. He was enjoying having the upper hand on Tom for once.

"You know what I mean. Who is she? What does she do? She looks like a model. What's she doing with you?" Tom was relentless.

"She is a flight attendant and since I am a Southern gentleman, I can't tell you what she does with me." Dave smiled mischievously.

Richard ended the conversation about Sharon, "She's Baby. You hear him on the phone with her at night every time we're on call."

After meeting Sharon, Tom's opinion of Dave improved considerably. It occurred to him, if Dave was with a woman like that, there had to be more to him than he originally thought. But it was Jason's opinion of Dave that really escalated. Jason considered women like Sharon out of reach, and his mind exploded when he realized an intern he worked with was with someone like her. After meeting Sharon, Jason mimicked Dave in every way, and Tom finally began to treat him like an equal. They became a real team at last, a tight functioning unit.

Near the end of the rotation, Dave's team was called to the ER for a patient with gunshot wounds to the abdomen. The man had been shot multiple times with a small caliber handgun at close range. The ER resident told them, "We caught this guy because both trauma rooms are tied up with cases, and we called you because none of the trauma staff are available. He has six entry wounds in his abdomen and only four exit wounds. He's lost a lot of blood and needs to go to the OR right away."

The resident continued, "He was shot by his wife, and she is in custody. The police told me she shot him because he kept coming home drunk, beating her, and having sex with her while he beat her. She bought a small caliber handgun, and told him if he did it again, she was going to kill him. He came in drunk, and she emptied the gun into his abdomen before he could touch her."

Tom told Richard and Dave to take the case so he could stay out to cover since both trauma teams and now one surgery team would be in surgery, but they knew Tom was just dodging another unpleasant case. The patient was a large Afro-American man whose name was Franklin. Dave examined him, and checked his x-rays and labs, while Richard wrote the admit note and pre-op orders.

Richard had started talking to Dave after meeting Sharon. "This is going to be an all-night sucker. We are going to find hole after hole in this guy's bowels and organs, then we have to go fishing for the two missing slugs in his back. I hate little handguns. I think they should be outlawed. People should only be able to buy big handguns, so when they shoot someone, they stay shot. All little handguns do is keep us up all night patching little holes."

Dave thought this was a novel way of looking at gun control and added, "Maybe all handguns should be outlawed?" The way Richard looked at him made him think he was going to stop talking to him again, but Richard had accepted him, liberal attitude and all.

"Jesus, Dave, I don't know where your head is sometimes, then I realize it is squarely up your ass. Where do you get these ideas from if you don't pull them out of your ass? Have you ever heard of the Second Amendment? Do you know what the Constitution is? You are a good guy, a good doctor, and I think you would make a hell of a fine surgeon, but you continue to amaze me with some of the things that come out of your mouth."

Richard was right, they were up all night, repairing Franklin's bowels and organs. Each time they ran his bowels or checked his organs, they found more holes. Finally, around dawn they began looking for the missing slugs. They found one embedded in his back muscles, which was easy to remove, but the other one was near the spinal cord, so they decided to leave it. They irrigate the man's abdomen with a lot of saline and closed. It was well into morning by the time Richard dictated the op note, Dave wrote post-op orders, and they left the man in the recovery room to go to breakfast.

When they got to the floor, Tom and Jason were waiting for them. Thinking Franklin was still in recovery, they all went down to see him, but he was not there. They checked back with the floor, but he was not there either, so Tom sent Jason down to the basement to check "Ground East" the morgue, but he was not in the morgue either. He was not in recovery, on the floor, or in the morgue. Tom began to panic because misplacing a patient was an unacceptable thing for a senior resident to do.

He asked Richard if the guy was doing well enough to have walked out of the hospital. Richard said he didn't think it was unlikely, so Tom called the attending to tell him they couldn't find one of their patients. The attending told him to call the city police and report the man missing, then call the hospital administrator and have him search for the patient. Tom's conversation with the city police left him embarrassed and humiliated. The officer he spoke to was more than a little critical of him losing a shooting victim.

The administrator could not find the patient either, so Tom called the attending again. He demanded Tom search the entire hospital, bed by bed if necessary, and God help him if he let a post-op patient walked out of the hospital status post multiple gunshot wounds.

Tom was already in trouble for an incident that took place before Dave joined the team. Richard told him. "Tom punched a Medicine resident. They argued about whether Medicine or Surgery should admit a patient and the Medicine resident got in Tom's face. He knocked the guy down with one punch and was almost dismissed from the program."

Richard and Dave had been on their feet all night, but they pulled themselves together to join Tom and Jason in floor-by-floor, room-by-room, bed-by-bed, station-by-station search of the hospital. It was early afternoon when Dave walked into the ICU and saw Franklin. He had been up all-night, so he was tired and a little less than cordial when he asked the nurse how the patient got to the ICU, and why the surgery team had not been informed he was there. The nurse was just as sharp with him when she told him she did not know how the patient got there. Someone had deposited him and left. Franklin didn't remember how he got to the hospital, much less how he got to the ICU. Tom got into a yelling match with the ICU charge nurse until they both calmed down long enough to transfer the patient to the surgery wards.

Dave finished his first surgery rotation conflicted. He had never considered becoming a surgeon, but now he felt a strong pull in that direction. He got an A in surgery in Med school, but he never considered it as a career choice. That was due to the fact he was not simply holding a retractor for someone else, but he was actually doing the surgery. Even when he assisted Richard, he did half of the procedure. Surgery was hands-on and physical, and he liked it the way he liked sports. Dave began to think he may have a decision to make about what he did for a residency.

Chapter 6

Halloween

Dave was going to the Halloween party as a pirate. His costume consisted of a black vest, red head scarf, mid-calf white duct pants, a wide black belt with a red sash that matched the head scarf under it, and a realistic-looking flintlock toy pistol to put in the belt. Sharon used black eye shadow to make his eyes look sinister, and red lipstick to draw a big anchor on his bare chest, then she sent him downstairs to wait for her.

She was going as a black cat, or a familiar. Her costume was a sheer black leotard with a long tail that curled up at the end. The leotard fit her like second skin covering her exquisite body from her ankles to her wrists, and six-inch black stiletto heels displayed her long dancer's legs to perfection. She put her lustrous hair up in a ponytail at the top of her head with a wide black band around its base, and she wore a black collar with a silver bell on it that matched the band around her neck. She used black eyeliner to make her eyes look cat-like, green eye shadow to accentuate their unusual color, and her lipstick was black. Her costume enhanced her natural beauty and transformed her into a living erotic fantasy.

It was a mild Indian Summer night with a bright full moon lighting up the landscape and a few small white puffy clouds drifting across the open sky. A perfect night for Halloween. They walked to the house next door and found Henry, Sherry, Mike, and Janice already in the front room. Janice was dressed as Dorothy from The Wizard of Oz and since she looked and acted like she was twelve years old; it was the perfect costume. Mike was not in a costume. Sherry was dressed as a hula dancer in a bikini with a grass skirt. She had flowers around her ankles, her wrists, and her head with several flower leis around her neck. Henry was dressed as a competitive swimmer, with a swim cap, swim goggles, a Speedo swimsuit, beach slip-ons, and nothing else.

"My God!" Mike blurted out. "Are you just painted?"

"Well, if you've got it, flaunt it. You've sure got it, and you sure are flaunting it." Sherry laughed, but it was a stilted laugh.

"I have on a black leotard, or a catsuit, only this one has a tail, like a cat, see." She showed them her tail.

"Hi, guys. I'm a pirate." Dave did a pose with his thumbs hooked in his belt.

"Really Dave? Do you think anyone is looking at you or cares that you are a pirate when they can look at Sharon in pretty much nothing but Sharon?" Henry's eyes, like Mike's, were fixed on Sharon as she looked over her shoulder at them holding her tail up.

"I thought Henry and I were being risqué wearing a Speedo and a bikini but Mike's right, you look like you have nothing on, and you have an incredible body. What I wouldn't give for your height. How tall are you with the stilettos, the hair, and everything?"

"I don't know; six inches of heels and the hair. I'm over five-nine in my bare feet."

"Man, that's a lot of...." Sherry frowned at Henry. "Cat ... I said cat."

Other people arrived, went to the dining room for beer or wine, put money in the bowl, and walked into the front room. The costumes were all exceptional and the party goers stayed in character to create a fantastical colorful mosaic of images.

Harvin let out a gorilla roar as he and Connie made their entrance. Connie was dressed in tight khaki short shorts, knee-high lace-up boots, a short-sleeve khaki shirt that was far too small, and an Australian bush hat pinned up on one side. The shirt could only be partially buttoned leaving a lot of Connie on display above the straining buttons. She was holding the leash of a gorilla with a studded collar. Harvin assumed all the attributes of a gorilla as he scurried along beside her.

"It is time for the costume contests. Find a place and we'll go through the categories." Harvin sat on his haunches picking at himself. "First category is sexist costume. If you want to participate, walk to the center of the room." He lay on his back holding his feet as Connie swung her arm around pointing at everyone as she went, but no one stepped out until she reached Sharon.

She leaned over to Dave and whispered, "Watch", stood up and cat walked to the center of the room amid whistles and lewd comments, turned back to face him with her feet apart and her hands on her hips, then shifted her weight from hip to hip, tossing her head from side to side with the hip action like a professional model. The wolf calls and whistles increased, including Harvin scurrying toward her sideways making his gorilla roar. Connie jerked on Harvin's leash, and he slunk back to sit at Connie's feet with his legs straight out. "It looks like we have a winner by acclamation."

Sharon stood in the middle of the room smiling at Dave, then she did her runway walk back, stood in front of him with her legs apart, bent at the waist, leaned over, put her hands on his shoulders, and whispered in his ear, "I did that for you." Her act had the effect on him she intended, but it also had the same effect on every other man in the room.

When she bent over Dave with her legs straight, they came to their feet yelling, including Henry, who then turned to her and said, "Jesus Christ, Sharon, where did that come from?" He could not believe the sophisticated, reserved Sharon he knew would put on such a performance.

Sherry huffed, "You know every woman in this room hates you now. How can the rest of us compete with you? With you and your six feet of … whatever … of cat? And all the men are picturing you … and believe me, you painted quite a picture for them to … imagine you in." Sherry was not pleased with Henry's behavior during Sharon's walk and posing.

"Well, that got the party started." Connie laughed. "Now, let's do the best costume. If you want to participate, walk to the center of the room, one at a time." Harvin sat up on his haunches to watch the parade of glitz and glitter. A woman covered in nothing but varying shades of green body paint, teased up dyed green hair, gossamer wings on her back, curved antennae on her head, and green slippers with turned up toes on her feet, won best costume. Harvin kept jumping up and down, running at her sideways, and roaring. The best couples costume was won by Connie and Harvin, the same way Sharon won, by acclamation.

After the costume contest, Connie led Harvin to the couch where Sharon, Sherry, Dave and Henry were sitting. "Don't stand right in front of me, Connie. If you pop a button, it will go right through me with all that force behind it."

"Very funny, Dave." Harvin started sniffing up Connie's leg. "I told you, Harvin, there is no way we were going to do it with you in that gorilla suit, so put that out of your head. Come on, I need something to drink after that." They followed Connie to the dining room, with Harvin sidling along beside her on his lease. Audrey and Jake were already in the dining room talking with Caroline and Ron.

Audrey was wearing her airline jacket with a black lace bra, black bikini panties, black garters, black nylons and stiletto heels. The jacket was a business suit coat, so it acted like a very low cut, short dress. Jake had on wing-tipped shoes, knee-high socks, black briefs, his airline jacket, and his pilot's cap with aviator sunglasses. "What did you guys think of the fairy? I thought Sharon was just painted until I saw the fairy. You could tell the difference."

"She wasn't completely naked. I talked to her. She had some kind of tape over her nipples and the business part of her who-haw." Ron had on a three-piece suit with a wolf mask on his head, wolf gloves on his hands, and wolf slippers on his feet.

Caroline was dressed as a sexy Little Red Riding Hood in a short petticoat skirt and a bib top with nothing on under it. "I bet it's going to hurt when she takes the tape off, but what kind of man do I have who says, who-haw instead of...."

Connie stopped Caroline. "We're not using that term tonight in deference to Sharon, who is a very tall one. But I have to agree. Is who-haw some kind of East Coast, Ivy League term; like Whiffenpoofs?"

Helen and her date walked up to the group. "Hi roommates, friends, and their significant others. This is Jackson. Jackson lives on the other side of the park and is some kind of consultant, but I have no idea what he consults on."

Jackson was a good-looking and well-built man in his late twenties. They were dressed as Helen of Troy and Paris, in lace up Greek sandals, short pleated white Greek skirts with garlands in their hair, and Jackson was bare chested. They all shook hands with Jackson and told him their names, except for Harvin, who sniffed at him. Jackson looked at the group. "I have been living on this park for years, and I never knew so many beautiful women lived in one house across from me."

"Down boy, Sherry and Connie don't live in our house, and my roommates are all in relationships. Sherry's boyfriend is the big one with nothing on and Connie is engaged to the gorilla." Harvin scurried at Jackson and roared.

"I am in a pulchritudinous paradise." Jackson oozed charm as he looked at Sharon. "What a night it would be if I could dance with you."

"If you have designs on the cat, forget it. After her performance, I am surprised she and the pirate haven't already swam upstream to spawn."

"Don't be mean, Helen." Sharon took Dave's arm.

Bob and Phil walked up to the group with their gift certificates. "Look at all the pretty people. You guys have no idea what an attractive group you are, and there is so much of you on display. Gay or straight, there is plenty of eye candy here for either." Bob was dressed as a Hobbit, with furry feet and all. Phil was in a Louie the Sixteenth costume. "Gorgeous, that little catwalk you did was something. You brought the house down and you certainly got all the men up", he paused "… on their feet." Phil laughed at his own joke.

"That walk was for my guy. I thought I made that obvious." She hugged Dave's arm to her.

"That's a pity," Jackson said, still looking at Sharon.

The speakers came alive, "It's time to get ready to commence to rock and roll people!"

Connie jerked on Harvin's leash. "You are not a gorilla, Harvin. You are a man, and if you don't stand up and act like one, you will be sleeping alone tonight."

Harvin stood up. "This is my true skin. When I put it on, I realized I have been a gorilla in a man's skin all this time. Now I'm a gorilla in a gorilla's skin. I'm in my true skin at last, besides if I take it off, I will be a naked ape."

"It's not your true skin, but I'm not dancing with you in nothing but your real true skin either, so keep it on. I will dance with a gorilla, but that's as far as it goes; do you understand?" Connie led Harvin to the front room on his leash.

Sharon backed out of the group, curled her index finger at Dave, put her hands close together above her head, closed her eyes, and started shifting her hips back and forth in time, as the music took control of her body. Dave yelled above the music, "It's going to be a hell of a night, Baby!"

"My God!" Jackson said as eyes followed Sharon's body.

"I am over here, and I told you to forget about her, she's taken." Helen replied.

"Take a look around. There isn't a guy here who isn't watching her," he shouted back and nodded at Mike, who was standing as if frozen with his eyes glued to Sharon, "and you can tell she likes to be watched. Look at her go."

Soon the house was packed with people dressed in all manner of costumes, stages of dress, or undress dancing in the dining room, the front room, the hall, and on the landing upstairs. Dave looked around. A gorilla was dancing next to him with Connie, who was on the verge of a major wardrobe malfunction; Henry, who was down to nothing but his Speedo, and Sherry in her bikini, her flowers and grass shirt long gone, were dancing behind Sharon. A big guy in combat boots, a male G-string, chains across his bare chest like bandoleers, and rabbit ears on his head was dancing on the other side of him with a woman in a G-string, heels, and smaller chains crossed between her bare breasts, and rabbit ears. Behind him a woman in nothing was dancing on the card table by herself. His brain was overloaded, as he watched the scene unfold around him. The front room looked like a living Hieronymus Bosch painting as an array of exotically costumed and bare skinned dancers shouted and gesticulated with their hands as the music blasted through them.

It went on song after song without a pause as more people gathered on the front porch and in the yard. Dave and Sharon were dancing close when T Rex's, Bang a Gong blasted out of the speakers. The song seemed to be an abstract description of his feelings for her, and he pulled her to him, kissing her passionately as it played. It all ended that way. Another song didn't start, instead Phil's voice came over the speakers. "OK, people, we have to wrap this up. We have to get everyone out of this house. The house has to be dark, quiet, and unoccupied except for the people staying here before the police start shutting down the parties. We can't have them coming in here with the air so heavy you can get high by just breathing, people getting it on in the back room, nude dancing, and all manner of recreational pharmaceuticals being passed around. It all has to stop. The music's over, and we are going to turn out the lights, so everyone needs to start moving out the door."

There was a lot of grumbling and some loud boos, but with no music and darkness, there was no reason to stay, so people began to leave. Bob got the couples dressed and out of the back room. George and his date, both dressed in roller derby costumes, cleared the landing on their way to George's room. Phil herded everyone out of the front room. Sam and Rachael, dressed as Robin Hood and Maid Mariam, moved them out of the dining room. They all keep everyone moving off the porch, out of the yard, and on to the street. Connie took Harvin's leash and led him up the stairs to his room saying, "No! I told you, I am not going to do it with you in that gorilla suit, so forget it!"

Sherry went to the dining room to find a lot more beer and white wine on ice in the cooler, unopened wine bottles of red wine on the table, and the bowl overflowing with bills. Henry stayed with Dave and Sharon in the front room. "Jesus Herman Christ, that was awesome. We tore it down; I mean, we tore it down!"

Jake, Audrey, Caroline, and Ron joined them. Jake was as animated as Henry. "Did you see all the people in nothing but body paint, not to mention those in nothing at all? Talk about your pagan rights on All Hollow's Eve."

Caroline asked Ron, "Did you ever go to a party like this back East at your Ivy League schools?"

"Are you kidding? I thought this was the Bible Belt, but that was pure debauchery at its finest."

Henry went to the dining room to find Sherry and the other three couples started back to the other house. Helen and Jackson caught up to them. "Who are you people? I have seen some crazy shit on this park, and some major parties, but nothing like this. Do a bunch of doctors live here? Is this the way doctors party?"

It was well after midnight when they said good night, planned to meet for breakfast the next morning, and went to their rooms. Sharon's costume, her catwalk, her dancing, the alcohol, the recreational substances; it all combined to produce a night of extremely erotic sex, so Sharon and Dave slept late and woke up a little hungover. Dave put on his pirate pants, Sharon put on her short robe, and they padded downstairs barefoot to the kitchen. They were greeted with applause. Dave looked at everyone. "What?"

"Not for you, for Sharon. She won a well-deserved title, representing our house." Helen held up her coffee cup in salute. "Let's hear it for our tall walking big black cat."

"Have you guys been up long?" Sharon ignored Helen's comments and sat down.

"Not long. Caroline and Ron were up first. We were waiting for you to start breakfast or to go out for brunch, but after last night, I don't think anyone is up for cooking or for getting dressed." Audrey, like all the women, had on a short robe.

"So, let's just have coffee and cereal. I'll get the cereal, milk, and bowls." Ron got up.

"I'll get some OJ and make toast." Jackson followed Ron.

Jake turned to Dave. "Man, that was one full tilt boogie last night. I am still trying to wrap my head around it."

Dave confessed, "I'm not sure everything I saw was real. I was wasted."

"You weren't the only one. There were some of the most messed up people I have ever seen in my life at that party, and there were a lot of who-haws, and ding-a-lings on full display. Did you see the couples dressed in latex, with whips and chains?" Jake shook his head.

Jackson chimed in from the toaster, "Halloween is always wild on the Park, but I have never seen anything like last night."

Once everything was ready and they were all seated, Helen looked around the table. "This is so much fun having everyone here. I wonder how many more times like this we'll have before every-thing changes."

Jackson had spent the night with Helen, and he was being included in the group, unlike the other men she dated. Sharon was at the house more than the other two women, and she hadn't seen him, and she wondered how long they had been seeing each other.

"This seems like as good a time as any to let everyone know Audrey and I are getting married in the Spring."

They all congratulated Audrey and Jake, but realized their announcement put a punctuation mark on what Helen said. They spent the rest of the morning talking and enjoying each other's company before splitting up for the rest of the day. Dave and Sharon went back to her room to shower before driving to Dave's apartment in separate cars. She was flying the next day, and he was starting the Surgery ER.

Chapter 7

The surgery ER

The Surgery ER rotation was twenty-four hours on and twenty-four hours off. He treated lacerations, abscesses, surgical abdomens, and mangled, broken body parts. At the end of a shift, he was covered with blood, pus, body fluids, and excretions.

He was sitting in the doctors' station drinking coffee one morning when a nurse walked by with a man with a bloody bandana wrapped around his head. The man told him he had been using a chainsaw, the saw kicked back, and cut his head. "No, I wasn't wearing any protective gear because I know how to handle a chainsaw and I don't need any. This was a freak accident. I just need a few stitches, not a safety lesion." Dave had the nurse help him as he unwrapped the bandana and washed the area with saline to expose the laceration. Once the wound was exposed, Dave realized he was looking at the man's brain through a wide groove in his scalp, skull, and dura. Another eight of an inch and the chainsaw would have taken a chunk out of his brain.

"Get me a stack of four by fours and some koban, then page Neurosurgery stat! Sir, you need to lie down right now. I need someone in here to start a large bore IV!" He got the man down despite his protests. "I don't need to lie down. All I need is a few stitches." Dave protected the wound, pressed the four by fours over it, and secured the dressing with the koban wrapped around the man's head. The neurosurgery resident showed up, Dave described the wound to him, and after he looked under the dressing, the resident whisked the man away to the OR amid continued protests that all he had was a cut that needed a few stitches. Dave sat back down in the doctor's station to take some deep breaths, try to get his heart rate down, and finish his

137

coffee. Most mornings were slow, then it picked up in the afternoon, and became busy at night.

But it was the Friday and Saturday night meetings of the city's knife and gun clubs that turned the ER into a living hell and demonstrated the violent, destructive nature of the human species to its fullest extent. The true nature of man is on display in its unvarnished form in the ER of a big city county hospital every weekend, and University Hospital was no exception. There are fights, muggings, and beatings with facial lacerations and fractures. Scalp lacerations, rib fractures, and other trauma that occurs when a weapon is involved. Then there are the stabbings and lacerations from knives, straight razors, and broken bottles. At times the department is full of the sounds of pain, and the cacophony of misery recurs every Friday and Saturday night without fail.

The weekend violence also has an audience: observers who relish watching the melodrama unfold from a front row seat. A road that leads into the hospital campus from the main street. On the right side of the road is the ambulance bay and on the other side is the entrance to the staff parking lot. The staff parking lot is on a hill that overlooks the ambulance bay, and every Friday and Saturday night groups of people gather on the hillside to watch the ambulances unload. With some trauma cases, the doctors and nurses are on the ambulance dock ready to begin treatment as soon as the ambulance doors open, and the crowd gets a good look at some real gore under the bright lights of the ambulance bay. The fact that the life-and-death struggle of one human being should be considered entertainment by another human being left Dave sickened by the depravity it demonstrated. The naïve, idealistic, young medical student who was out to save the world, was being morphed into a cynical, disillusioned young intern who was not sure the world was worth saving. In the surgery ER he was seeing the world through a very dark lens; the lens of violence.

But one foggy morning, the hillside revealed another side of humanity. As the long nights of November dragged on, the mornings became colder and foggier. On this particular morning the fog was so dense Dave could barely see to drive and when he arrived, he could only see dull smudges from the lights of the ambulance bay and fuzzy red blurs from the ambulances themselves. He got out of his car and heard a hauntingly beautiful voice floating on the fog singing the spiritual, Just a Closer Walk with Thee. He knew the voice was coming from the hillside, but he could not see anyone, and the sunrise added a dull homogeneous glow to the fog, so it seemed as if the voice was disembodied, without a source, and emanating from the fog itself. The singer had perfect pitch and the warm melodious voice of a black gospel singer. It was so filled with sorrow and emotion, it tore at his very soul, and when she let her voice soar on the chorus, "Oh Lord let be", it cut through the fog like a knife that cut through his heart. He stood there engulfed in the pain of the voice and shaken to his core by its effect on him. How could humans produce something that beautiful, soulful, and emotional yet also produce the devastation he was about to deal with in the ED? Yet, he knew it was the very man-made horror he was about to walk into that produced the beauty and emotion in the voice. That dichotomy left him confused. The fact that man, the most violent and destructive species on the planet, the homo species that survived to evolve because it wiped out all the other hominin species, could produce such beautiful soulful music was difficult for him to reconcile.

The realization that no one was immune to the violence had already been demonstrated to him in crystal-clear fashion by his interaction with the biker in the Medicine ER, but that fact was further reinforced one night in mid-November. He had finished suturing a laceration and was on his way to the doctors' station to write his note when two city police officers came through the Surgery ER doors. "Close and secure these doors. No one leaves this room. You are to shelter in place." The two police officers stationed themselves on each side of the doors with their weapons drawn.

Tom approached one of the police officers. "What's up?"

The officer responded. "A man tried to murder his wife, but she survived and was brought here for treatment. He showed up later at the triage desk asking for her. We think he is armed and is trying to find her to finish her off."

Tom called the staff together. "Let's get all the patients as far back from the doors as possible and put any empty gurneys, Mayo stands, chairs, or anything else we can find between them and the doors. Once we get everyone relocated, we need to keep taking care of our patients. Richard, find out where the wife is and what's going on." Richard called the Trauma charge nurse, and she told him the patient had been taken to the OR.

"OK, everybody, just stay calm and do your job. We're well protected and we'll be fine. Let's get back to work." Tom was known for his fearlessness when he played football at the University of Texas.

After some time, one of the police officers informed them it was over. "We got him," and the two officers left. Later, they heard there had been a gunfight in the hall outside the OR and the husband had been killed. The doctors operating on the wife could hear the gunshots, but they kept operating trying to save the woman's life with the firing going on just outside the operating suite doors.

The last case in the Surgery ER that left an indelible impression on him occurred the day before Thanksgiving. Sherry gave Henry an ultimatum on Thanksgiving; either take their relationship to the next level or move back into the park house. Henry moved back to the park house the day after Thanksgiving and Sherry moved on.

The med students and the other flight attendants were going home for Thanksgiving. Sharon and Dave were having Thanksgiving with Bob and Phil. Sharon knew her mother would be lonely without her, but if she went home, Dave would be alone since he was off on Thanksgiving Day. Thanksgiving is a family holiday so the urges she fought so hard to control troubled her again, but she pushed those feelings down and told herself she was happy just the way they were.

He caught a patient late that night who was brought in by the city police. He had worked out a system with Jason to ease the workload, speed up the flow, and allow for some teaching. They saw patients together. If Jason could handle the case alone, Dave moved on to the next one, but if it was beyond Jason's capabilities, he helped Dave with the work-up and treatment.

The patient was an Afro-American man with his hands and feet shackled to a gurney who had been savagely beaten. His eyes were swollen, his nose was crooked, his lips were split, and he had multiple burst wounds on his scalp. There were three police officers with him, and one of them spoke to Dave. "We need him treated and cleared medically as soon as possible, so we can take him to jail."

Dave had seen injured patients who needed to be treated and cleared so they could be incarcerated before, but he had never seen one this savagely beaten. "What did he do?" The man reeked of alcohol, urine, and feces.

The officer responded, "He murdered his wife, then he killed one of our officers who was responding to the domestic disturbance call." He looked at the other two officers. "He resisted arrest and we had to subdue him."

Dave checked the man neurologically, examined his chest and abdomen, and instructed Jason to, "Wash and get some pressure on the scalp wounds to control the bleeding, then get a tech to cut his clothes off and clean him up. Once that's done, call me and we can check him carefully before we send him to X-ray. Order a skull series, rib series, and facial bones. When he gets back from x-ray, call ENT to take care of his nose and any other facial fractures, then we'll suture his wounds. Tell the radiologist we need a reading right away." He spoke to the police officers. "I'm sorry about your officer. I'll do everything I can to get this man treated and cleared. Is there anything else I can do to help?"

The officer shook his head. "No, but you can imagine what it means for us to lose one of our own."

Dave told Jason, "Stay with this patient and ride herd on everyone to get him out of here ASAP. Page me when everything is done."

After a thorough exam and x-rays, ENT took care of the man's fractured nose, then Jason and Dave sutured his wounds with one of them working on each side of the man's face and scalp, and when the wounds were closed, Dave signed off on the patient clearing him for incarceration.

He had finished seeing another patient and was walking back to the doctor's station when he was met by the officer who had spoken to him before. "We need you back, Doc." The police officer led him back to the man, who was still shackled to the gurney. Both the man's eyes were completely swollen shut, his bandaged nose was smashed again, he had new wounds and some of the sutured ones were split open. He had been severely beaten again and there was a new police officer with him who spoke. "He tried to escape."

Dave looked at the four police officers. "We spent hours neglecting other patients to take care of this man so you could get him out of here as quickly as possible, now we are going to have to do it over again while other patients wait. If you are going to do anything else to him, do it now, so we don't have to do our work all over a third time."

The new police officer stepped up to Dave and pointed his finger at his chest. "This nigger killed my partner, and he is getting what he deserves: you'll do what I tell you to do, as many times as I tell you to do it, understand!"

"No, I won't. Your authority ends at the medical care of this patient and my authority begins there. He is under my care, in my emergency room." Dave looked with disdain at the finger the police officer was pointing at his chest.

The policeman's face went a vivid red, his eyes became menacing, and the veins in his forehead bulged as he jabbed his finger into Dave's chest. "Look, you nigger lover!"

Tom walked up because he heard the shouting. "Knock that shit off and I mean, now! I think it would be a good idea for you guys to get this officer out of here before I call our security and have him thrown out. We'll take care of this patient again after we clear the backlog caused by putting his case above our other patients. If you have a problem with that, give me your captain's name. I'll call him and discuss it with him. I'm sure he will be pleased to know how one of his officers is conducting himself in a hospital ER in front of a lot of witnesses, no matter how distraught that officer is." Tom was big, loud, and imposing, so when the police officer confronting Dave turned to Tom, the other two officers intervened, took him by the arms, and hustled him out of the ER despite his protest.

The remaining officer who had been talking to Dave apologized to Tom. "I'm sorry, but he just lost his partner so give him a break."

"I understand, but Dr. Cameron didn't kill his partner and he is doing everything he can to help. Attacking a physician who is only trying to do his job is not going to bring his partner back. We'll get your prisoner taken care of, but we have other people to care for, too. Go ahead with your other patients Dr. Cameron, you can take care of this man again when you're caught up."

"Jason can take care of him. He knows what to do because it is simply a repeat of the work-up and treatment we just did." Jason nodded. He had been watching the whole exchange wide eyed.

Tom looked at the officer. "If I were you, I would thank Dr. Cameron profusely for going out of his way to help you because he is going to have Jason write a follow-up note on this patient and what happened here. That note will be evidence in the man's chart, so how he writes the note will determine if that officer keeps his badge or not. This is not the streets, and you are not dealing with criminals here. This is a hospital ER, and you are dealing with dedicated professionals. How dare one of you treat one of them that way? If one of you ever insults or threatens one of my doctors again, you will see me on the six o'clock news publicly filing charges against him after the hospital administrator calls the mayor. Make sure your captain knows that. And one more thing, don't think you can beat a prisoner in this ER again, no matter what he has done, and make sure the rest of your colleagues know that, too. Is that all clear?" The officer nodded.

Jason sutured the wounds, ENT put the man's nose back in place, and all the x-rays were negative. Dave was writing his note when the first police officer spoke to him. "Look Doc, he's not a bad guy. He lost control because this guy killed his partner. Don't ruin his career because he was reacting like any of us would under the same circumstances."

"That man is emotionally unstable, and you know it. He was coming after me. What's going to happen to the next black man he arrests? What's going to happen to the next white man, like me, who crosses him? I looked the other way when you brought this man in badly beaten because of the very reasons you just mentioned. You want me to look the other way when he is beaten while he is shackled to a gurney in the hospital ER hours after the shooting? I'm writing this up exactly as it happened. I would advise you and the other two officers to get on the right side of this while you can. My first note doesn't mention anything but the injuries, so you guys are not implicated in any way in how he presented to the ER, but the second note will outline just what happened here. That officer is psychologically unfit to be carrying a badge and a gun."

"Have it your way Doc, but recently some of our guys protected some of your guys." The officer pressed Dave.

"And we're grateful, but he is out of control, and you know it. What if I protect him; will you take responsibility for his future actions? I'll be happy to write a note stating that you personally reported to me that a man whose hands and feet were shackled to a gurney in a hospital ER had to be beaten senseless to prevent him from escaping. You want me to do that?" Dave looked at the officer with a questioning expression.

"I guess not." The officer replied and hung his head.

"Look, I'm sorry about your murdered colleague. I'm sorry about a lot of the things I have to deal with in this ER. But it's my job to deal with them no matter how awful they are. It's your job to prevent them from happening. Believe me, I know that it is a tough job because I see the fallout from it every day. You guys go in harm's way to protect the rest of us, but that's your job. It certainly isn't part of your job to add to the carnage, like that officer did." Dave walked away to find Tom and thank him. Tom was a jerk, but he always came through and handled any situation correctly.

Dave finished his shift and drove home to get some sleep before Thanksgiving dinner, but he did not sleep well. His two experiences in the ED, coupled with the gun fight outside the OR had unnerved him considerably. He had been in danger twice and one of those times it was from someone who was supposed to be protecting him. That gnawed at him as he drove to Sharon's.

Dave and Sharon were from Southern families that dressed for Thanksgiving and Christmas dinners, so he wore a suit, and she wore a conservative dress. They rang the doorbell at Bob's and Phil's house around four in the afternoon.

Phil answered the door. "My God, Ken and Barbie are here to have Thanksgiving with us."

"Ken has dark hair and Barbie is blond." Sharon walked past Phil into the living room.

Phil stood at the door and looked at Dave. "Don't tell me you two have had a lover's quarrel."

Sharon stopped, turned, and apologized for being abrupt. "I'm sorry Phil, but I usually go home for Thanksgiving dinner to be with my mother, and I feel guilty about leaving her alone."

Bob joined them. "Why didn't you invite her to have Thanksgiving dinner with us?"

"No offense guys, but I have a big picture of that." They all walked into the living room to join Sharon. "Mom, why don't you have Thanksgiving dinner with me, the intern I'm sleeping with, and our two gay friends."

Phil motioned them toward the couch. "I take it mom is old-school?"

"She is beyond old-school. Victorian is more like it. She sees herself as Southern gentry and has visions of me marrying someone from a prominent old Southern family. All I need to do to complete her disappointment in me is to tell her I am sleeping with a guy with long blond hair and hanging out with a gay couple."

"I will be back with some bourbon, and we will wash those blues away." Bob left.

"Dave, you don't look happy either. It's Thanksgiving. You especially have a great deal to be thankful for." Phil indicated Sharon with a glance.

"I'm sorry, Phil. I've been spending too much time with the fine citizens of our fair city getting a close-up view of how they treat one another, and it is disheartening."

Bob returned with four bourbons. "Wrap your lips around these, and I guarantee it will lift your spirits." When they all had a glass, Bob lifted his. "Happy Thanksgiving."

"Is there anything in this, or is it just a big glass of bourbon?" Sharon said in a hoarse voice.

"Big damn glass of bourbon, and here's to it." He raised his glass again and drank so they took a second drink. After two big shots of bourbon, the mood lightened.

Dinner was excellent with traditional turkey and dressing with cranberry sauce, sweet potatoes, mashed potatoes with gravy, plus pumpkin pie for dessert. They drank a bottle of wine with dinner then Bob brought brandy out after dinner. They drank brandy and talked as the earth rotated into evening, then into the darkness of night. With their side of the earth hidden from the bright starlight of the sun, they went back to Sharon's house and went to sleep. He slept better next to her, but he was still troubled.

Dave's next rotation was the Trauma Service. His surgery team would become Trauma 2. His last day in the Surgery ER was a day off and they spent the afternoon sitting together in one of the bean bags talking about their future plans.

"I'm going to file my applications for residency, and you should apply to the MBA programs. It will take some time to get everything together, do the paperwork, request transcripts and recommendations, so you should get started this month."

She drifted on a dream of her future as he talked. He would be a doctor, she could have a career, and they would live in Northern California. They would have money with both their incomes, so they could go to Europe and spend time on the beaches of Hawaii, drive nice cars, and have a home she would decorate with original art and stylish furniture. She was so lost in her fantasy she didn't hear anything he said until, "So, what do we do for the rest of this afternoon?"

She didn't answer because as she came back from her fantasy it occurred to her that she had undergone a fundamental change. She never had plans for her future. She had been a beautiful woman getting by on her looks and running or flying away from her past, but now she was going as far as her intelligence and abilities could take her. She wanted the dream she had just dreamed and the future she had just fantasized about, and she was motivated to achieve it with a longing like nothing she had experienced before. These feelings were new to her, but they came together for her as she looked at him. He did this to her. He taught her the pleasures of sex, he restored the joy of dance for her, he showed her how wonderful a caring relationship could be. More importantly, he had helped her find herself. She cradled his head to her breast and hung on to him without saying a word. She didn't know how to express how she felt, so she simply clung to him in silence.

Dave looked into her eyes and lost himself in her eyes as he always did. "Is this what you want to do for the rest of the afternoon and tonight?"

She smiled. "Pretty much." They didn't get dressed and they didn't leave the apartment until the next morning when they both went to work the next day.

Chapter 8

The Trauma Service

His team had developed a bit of a swagger because they were one of the best, if not the best, surgery team on the house staff. Shifts on the Trauma Service went from seven AM until seven AM with the followed by twenty-four hours off. The teams never left the ED during a shift but waited in the trauma call room for announcements alerting them to incoming patients. They slept there on the couches and ate from the machines in the break room. During the down times, they read or napped. There were extended periods of boredom interspersed with intense, stressful periods of frantic activity.

They took on car accidents, industrial accidents, gunshot wounds, and a whole meridian of broken, torn, and mangled body parts; from severed or partially severed limbs, to gashed or ripped open abdomens and chests, to smashed heads and crushed extremities. It was bloody, ghastly work. Trauma Surgery required steady nerves and unwavering courage. It was not for the timid or weak minded.

They were sitting in the call room on a Saturday night and Dave was talking to Sharon amid a considerable number of lascivious background comments questioning his manhood, extolling their own manly prowess, and calling on her to abandon him for one of them, when the overhead came alive. "Trauma One and Trauma Two, four, repeat four ambulances five minutes out with four victims, repeat four victims, with multiple injuries due to MVA."

They ran to the unit and quickly prepared the room for two patients. They barely had everything in place when the doors burst open, the ambulance crews ran in with two gurneys, and the patients were transferred to the operating tables amid the organized chaos that invariably precedes the care of severally injured patients. As the ambulance crews gave their reports, the nurses started cutting the victim's clothes away. "My God, their babies!" The first patient was a very pretty young blond girl, not more than sixteen or seventeen. Dave looked over at the other table and saw another young girl about the same age with dark hair. He quickly intubated the blond girl, then moved to the other table to intubate the second girl. The dark-haired girl's abdomen was grotesquely distended, and they were both very pale. The anesthesiologist arrived and put lines in the girls, while Jason and the charge nurse started fluids. He checked the girl's pupils and both girls were reactive, but the nurse reported they had no blood pressure. The anesthesiologist got both girls on ventilators with 100% oxygen and started typed blood.

Dave joined Richard as he opened the dark-haired girl's abdomen and blood gushed out. "Suction and retraction. She has a ruptured spleen. I need to isolate the splenic artery and clamp it." They got the splenic artery clamped, but the massive bleeding continued, and more blood was coming out than could be pushed in. "She has a lacerated liver; we need to clamp the hepatic artery, and then I can get the bleeding controlled. More suction." They clamped the hepatic artery, but the bleeding continued. "More suction and more retraction." Richard continued to search for another source of the bleeding. "My God, she has massive vascular damage. We can't control this and there is no way to repair it."

The anesthesiologist said in a matter-of-fact voice, "She is fixed and dilated."

The charge nurse added, "She has no pressure or pulse."

Richard looked at Dave. "She is gone."

Richard went to the other table to join Tom and Jason. Tom had made an incision in the blond girl's chest and his hand was inside her chest cavity rhythmically squeezing her heart, as blood and fluids were pushed through the IVs.

"She has no pulse or pressure and her CVP (venous pressure measured through a central line) is zero. Your compressions aren't doing any good because she is not filling between compressions. Let's look. Jason retract. Tom, take your hand out." Richard pulled the incision apart as Jason retracted. Blood poured out, "Suction and more retraction. Look Tom, all of her pulmonary vessels are torn. We are just putting blood in her chest cavity. There is no blood return to her heart."

"She is fixed and dilated." the anesthesiologist added.

"She is gone."They let the incision go and pulled the retractor out as the wound closed, oozing blood.

Tom exploded, "God damn it! God damn it!" He stormed out of the room.

"They both had lethal injuries. There was nothing we could do. I'll pronounce them and write the note. I don't think Tom is very functional right now. Dave, check with the triage desk and see about the families. Come get me when you know what's going on out there."

Dave looked at the scene and it was burned into his memory for the rest of his life. All the lines and endotracheal tubes were pulled, and the beautiful blond girl looked like she was sleeping with a calm expression on her angelic face: the only sign that anything was wrong was a red line under her left breast. But the dark-haired girl's abdomen was gaped open with blood covering her, the table, and the floor. Her head was back with her eyes open in an expression of horror. Dave couldn't look away from the scene as he stood there with emotion welling up in his chest.

He struggled with what it meant for these two young girls to be snuffed out in the Spring of their young lives. They would never go to more proms or homecoming dances, they would never graduate from high school, go to college, experience love, get married, and have children. The old questions exploded in his head. He didn't ask where a benevolent, caring God was in all this. He had given up on that question. But he did ask, as he always did whenever he was confronted with death: what is life? Is there more to life than complicated electrophys-iologic processes and organic chemical reactions? If there is, what is it, what is the life force? *These girls were here and now they're gone. Where did they go? Where did their essence go? Did it just drift off into the ether? Did they simply return to stardust? Is there really a soul? Do all living things have a soul? Are we all just a magical collection of stardust that ignites into life briefly then returns to the elements we are made of, or is there more to it than that?* Death was always too much for Dave, and every time he confronted it, he failed to comprehend it or process it.

He went to the ED waiting room and the triage nurse pointed him to two highway patrol officers who told him they had notified the four kids' parents of the accident. The other trauma team's senior resident told him one boy was DOA, the second boy was brain dead, on life support, and he was waiting for the parents' consent to pull the plug on him. Dave asked a highway patrol officer to come get him in the trauma call room when the girls' parents arrived.

The incident had affected Dave deeply but not as deeply as it affected Tom, who was sitting in the trauma call room covered in blood with his gown and gloves still on. "I had her little heart in my hand. I should have been able to do something. I held her life in my hand, and I let it slip away." He looked down at his bloody gloved hands like Lady Macbeth.

"She had lethal wounds, there was nothing you could've done." Richard tried to console him, but Tom just kept staring at his bloody hands. Dave finally broke his trance. "The parents of both girls are on their way in."

"Dave, can you and Richard handle them? I need to get cleaned up." He headed for the locker room to wash up and change his scrubs. Tom blamed himself for the young girl's death and he was never the same. Her death humbled him. He had always been a good surgeon, he had always handled things well and done the right thing, but he was also arrogant and cocksure about his abilities. The experience transformed him from simply being a good surgeon, to being a good, caring doctor. Unfortunately, a beautiful young girl had paid a terrible price to facilitate his transition.

A highway patrol officer appeared at the door. "They're all here."

"You take the dark-haired girl's parents. What was her name? I'll take the blond girl's parents. No details, just the facts. They had lethal injuries. That's all. Nothing more. Spare them any of the particulars." Dave went out to do one of the most unpleasant tasks he would do during his internship.

They talked to the parents then got an on-call psychiatrist to see them and Richard contacted the chaplain to comfort them. The poor parents were shattered and decimated with grief. That was another thing Dave would never forget, their destitute cries of anguish.

The four kids were juniors in high school, and they had gone to the city to see a movie. On their way home, a drunk driver careened into their car, sending it over the median into the oncoming traffic where an eighteen-wheeler hit them broadside. The drunk driver didn't have a driver's license because it had been suspended for previous DUIs. His car skidded to a stop on the shoulder, and he was unhurt. The driver of the eighteen-wheeler seemed out of it when the highway patrol questioned him, so they searched his cab and found amphetamines.

The highway patrol officer said the truck was fully loaded and probably going close to ninety, so it was like the kid's car was hit by a freight train. That's what burst the girl's internal organs and ruptured their blood vessels: their bodies literally exploded from the impact. The emotion of the whole incident coupled with what happened to the girls' bodies sickened Dave. His brain cried out, and it was all he could do to keep from throwing up.

He went back to the trauma call room and buried the whole incident in the graveyard where he buried all the other damaging things he had experienced during his internship. But the graveyard was getting crowded, and it was becoming harder to keep the ghosts at bay. His emotions were being turned off in order for him to survive the psychological trauma he was being subjected to. The question was, would they turn back on of their own accord, or would he be able to turn them back on once his training was over?

There was another incident that left an indelible impression on him during his trauma rotation, but it had nothing to do with trauma surgery. After his team stabilized and transferred a patient to Orthopedics, Dave saw an overweight Afro-American woman in the hall, "We're finished in Trauma Two and it needs to be cleaned."

The black woman turned slowly to look at him. "And who might you be?"

"I am Dr. Cameron." He realized from the way she acted and spoke she was not a member of the cleaning crew, but it was too late

She looked Dave up and down with disdain. "I am the chief resident of thoracic surgery, and I am on my way to see a GSW to the chest, not to clean a room."

His face colored. "The GSW is in Trauma One."

The black woman scowled at him. "You think I don't know that? Do you think I am stupid because I am Black?"

"No. I'm sorry." Dave was more than embarrassed now, he was worried. Subspecialty chief residents worked directly with attendings.

"Are you now? You know what you are? You're a Southerner white boy who is the product of his upbringing and environment. That's why you assumed I was a cleaning lady. Have you ever talked to a Black woman who wasn't a maid in your house or some other white person's house? No, I doubt it. I need to get a bullet out of a man's chest now, so I don't have any more time to waste on you and your inherent racism." She continued to Trauma One.

He stood watching her walk away as if he had been struck by a thunderbolt. What she said was true. Both his mother and grandmother had Afro-American maids. Even in medical school he didn't talk to any of the Afro-American women there. All the way through school he had stuck to a close set of friends that mirrored him in every way. As a result, a mindset had been programmed into him, and it remained rooted in his perceptions.

No wonder racism is such a problem. Add in man's inherent tribalism, mix it with xenophobia, stir it with bigotry, and what you get is a complex toxic problem with no simple solution. Racism is something that will take fundamental changes in the whole milieu of the entire human experience to resolve. That conclusion left Dave with a hollow feeling. He was willing to try to correct his inherent racial bias, but how many others weren't even willing to address their mind set: much less try to change it. The believing brain believes what it wants to believe, and seldom listens to a point of view that doesn't coincide with its already preconceived deductions.

The Christmas season came and went for Dave without much fanfare. He and Sharon drove around the park area looking at the decorated houses, they had dinner in the city and walked around afterwards looking at the decorations in the store windows, and they shopped at the mall near his apartment to enjoy the decorations there, but that was it. It was his first Christmas away from home and he spent it in the hospital. Sharon was not going to leave her mother alone at Christmas, so she went home. She was flying and he was working the day she came back, so they didn't see each other for four days, the longest they had been apart since the night they met.

They exchanged gifts before she left. Dave gave her a bracelet with a heart on it engraved with the word "Forever". She gave Dave a nice leather case with his initials on it. Bob and Phil had people over for drinks on Christmas Eve, but everyone was gone except Dave, Mike, and Henry. Henry and Mike walked over together, and Dave drove in from his apartment. Rachael and Sam were there too, but no one else. He stood around talking and drinking Champagne for a few hours then went home to get a good night's sleep before his shift on Christmas Day. Sharon called later to wish him a Merry Christmas, but he was depressed without her, and hearing her voice only made it worse.

The ED was busy on Christmas, but there was only one trauma case, and it went to the other Trauma team, so Dave's team hung around in the trauma call room listening to Christmas music playing on the overhead. They slept through the night on the couches, and he went home to spend the next day without her. She called again that night, but they didn't talk long. It was absolutely the worst Christmas of his life.

His last day on the Trauma service was also his last day on the Surgery service. Tom told Dave he was proud to have had him on his team, even though he was a panty waist liberal. He took his hand firmly, "Take care of yourself and take care of Baby. I wish you both all the best." High praise from the "new" Tom. Richard took his hand, "You're going to start your applications soon. Think about doing Surgery and think about doing it here. I think you would make a fine surgeon. You have the nerve, you have excellent hands, and you can perform under stress. Tom and I will support your application." Dave valued Richard's respect more than anyone he worked with during his internship. Jason thanked him and said goodbye. Dave thought about the kid who fainted in the ER on their first call and what a solid, steady man he was now.

He drove home thinking about the last three months. His Surgery rotation had been tough on him. He had suffered emotionally and physically, yet a part of him would miss the drama and intensity. He had always been a bit of an adrenaline junkie, but it wasn't something he wanted to do for the rest of his life. He shifted his thoughts to the New Year's Eve party and Sharon. His next rotation was OB/GYN ER, but first there was the party and night with the woman he loved. He buried the bodies deeper, pushed the ghosts back into the graveyard, and his mood brightened thinking about Sharon; her beauty, her warmth, her intellect, everything about her. It was New Year's Eve, and he was halfway through his internship.

Chapter 9

New Year's Eve

Dave didn't want to drive on New Year's Eve after what he saw during his rotation on the Trauma service, so he booked a room at the Hotel. He wore his black suit and Sharon wore an elegant red satin dress she bought in New York for the occasion. Her hair was curled into large deep ringlets that flowed over her shoulders and down her back, her makeup was alluring with red lipstick that matched the color of the dress, and green eyeshadow that matched her eye color. The smell of her perfume was heady, and she had used a fragrant body lotion that left her skin soft, moist, and sparkling with glitter. In a word, she was exquisite.

After he dealt with the valet parking attendant and a bellman for the bags, he entered the hotel lobby to find her surrounded by three men. They were animated, all talking at once, and gesturing with their hands as they pressed close to her, competing for her attention. She was shaking her head, saying "no," and laughing as they maneuvered with each other to get closer to her. He didn't hesitate, but barged briskly through the men, elbowed them aside, and offered her his arm.

As they walked away, he asked, "Who were those guys? What did they want?"

She acted nonchalant. "Some German businessmen trying to do a little business with me. They got into a bidding war for me, and the last offer was very tempting, plus the guy was kind of cute. I could have done some business with him, had a good time, and made a lot of money tonight."

He stopped, "What!"

"They were trying to buy me for a night of passion." she teased him. "What can you offer me for … what did one of them say … I know: a good time' tonight?"

He looked back at the three men, who were still watching Sharon. "What!" He turned on them.

She pulled him back to her. "Calm down. You get so jealous. But let this be a lesson to you: don't leave me alone in a hotel lobby. I might change professions." She smiled mischievously.

The three men saw him move toward them scowling and walked away quickly. "Did you tell them you weren't an escort, and you were waiting for me?"

"Yes, but they were a little drunk, their English wasn't that good, and they were very excited about me. I know now what a night of sex with me is worth, and I don't think you can afford me. In fact, I think you owe me a hell of a lot of money." She continued to tease him.

"I'm not letting you out of my sight again tonight." He knew how desirable she was, but it never occurred to him that another man might try to buy her. The fact that a man would think he could purchase her like a commodity unnerved him considerably. It demonstrated to him there were wealthy men in the world who lived by a code of conduct vastly different from his naïve values.

They checked in and the desk clerk gave them a room upgrade, leering at Sharon the whole time. He gave their room number to the bell captain, and they made their way to the ballroom where a line of attractive, well-dressed couples were paying, receiving glasses of Champagne, and wristbands at a table by the ballroom door. They found Connie, Audrey, Harvin, and Jake in the line.

"Where is Henry? He is the one who picked this party and made the reservations. Was he still at the house when you left, Harvin?" Dave looked up and down the line.

"I haven't seen Henry for a while. He met with Sheffield to go over his plan to apply for a fellowship in Infectious Disease and Sheffield arranged for him to meet with someone from the Immunology Department at the University. I haven't seen him since." Harvin looked around. "There he is."

Henry, in a perfectly tailored suit, strode toward the group with a very tall blond woman on his arm. She was dressed in a silver cocktail dress and as they got closer, Dave saw she was hauntingly beautiful. Her hair was so blond it was almost white, her eyes were light blue, and she was slim but also fit.

"Sigrid, these are my friends. Sharon, Connie, Audrey, Dave, Harvin, and Jake. Sigrid finished her PhD in Immunology at the University of Copenhagen this year and is working on a joint research project between her university and ours. She hasn't been in the States long or met many people, so I asked her to join us tonight."

Sigrid released Henry's arm, stepped forward, and offered her hand to each of them in turn. "I have heard a great deal about all of you and I am so pleased to meet you." Her English was perfect with a Danish accent that made her sound decidedly sexy. Dave took her hand. *She's a lab rat like Henry, a big, beautiful lab rat.* The women in Henry's life all fit a mold: cute, rich, well bred, sophisticated, and deferential to Henry. Sherry had been a perfect example of Henry's type. Sigrid was tall with a universal beauty. She was the product of a social democracy, and he could tell immediately she wasn't deferential to anyone. He thought at another time in history she would have been a famous shield maiden. She was the very embodiment of a Valkyrie.

Dave smiled and almost laughed out loud as he remembered what Henry said to him about Sharon. *Touché my friend. You looked into the pool of the other person and saw yourself.* Henry took charge when they reached the reception table and paid for all of them. "It's my party." They found their table in the ballroom, but Henry stopped them from sitting down, and raised his glass, "Here's to us, to our friendship. May we continue to share nights like this for many more New Years to come." They clinked glasses, took a sip of Champagne, and sat down.

Sigrid looked around the table. "I want to thank all of you for allowing me to join you tonight, Skol." She raised her glass to them and took a sip of her Champagne.

Jake was sitting next to her. "Sigrid, tell us how you met Henry, and Henry, I doubt you're simply being a good Samaritan to a beautiful, lonely Danish girl who is new to our country?"

Audrey was on the other side of Jake. "He's right, are you two dating? I am sorry, but as Henry's friends it's only natural we are going to grill you a little."

"Henry said you are all close friends, there are actually more of you in this 'gang', and that the couples here tonight are all lovers." Dave saw a fierce intelligence behind her pale blue eyes that were now sparkling with mirth. "And he told me you two made love at first sight."

"No Sigrid, I said they fell in love at first sight." Henry tried to correct her.

"No, Sigrid is right. We did make love at first sight. Everyone knows that. We fell in lust at first sight." They were all happy and young with their lives spread out before them waiting to be lived: it was New Year's Eve, the night to leave the past behind and celebrate the future.

"And are you still in lust?" Sigrid continued to look at them with her pale blue eyes that seemed to see everything clearly.

Sharon gave Dave an intimate look. "Little bit."

Sigrid looked at Henry with the same intimate look and touched his arm. "Is that the way it is with you Americans? You fall in lust?" The look Sigrid gave Henry told Sharon everything she needed to know about their relationship, and the way Henry looked back generated enough heat, Sharon could feel it across the table.

Still looking at Henry, Sigrid continued, "The leader of my team told me I had to meet with this American doctor who wanted to know about Immunology research." Sigrid looked back at them. "I was very annoyed. I had a lot of work to do, and I did not have time to waste on some doctor who was too dumb to know how Immunology related to

Infectious Disease. I had to set aside a whole afternoon to meet with him on a day he chose because of his schedule, with no regard for my schedule. I had to meet with this moron when I was already behind in my work, so I decided to be unpleasant to him, end the meeting early, and get back to my work as quickly as possible. I was even more annoyed when this tall, handsome, charming man shows up, and distracts me to the point I find myself not wanting to be unpleasant to him and go back to work. We talked into the evening about how to deal with virus strains that attenuate so quickly they don't lend themselves to an immunological form of treatment. We argued because he is very arrogant and thinks he knows everything."

Harvin interrupted. "I'm shocked. Shocked to hear that Henry is arrogant."

Dave added. "I'm more shocked to hear that Henry thinks he knows everything."

Sigrid laughed, "It is obvious you both know him well. It got late, and we were still talking, so he asked me to go to dinner with him."

Harvin continued to goad Henry, "Henry, you sly dog, you wooed her with immunologically resistant, attenuating virus strains."

Dave followed with, "How could she resist the temptation of doing a double-blind study with you on how a virus strain's protein coat affects its virulence?"

"Very funny. You two think you are so funny." But Henry was smiling, and it was obvious he was enjoying himself immensely.

Sigrid addressed Dave. "What did you talk to Sharon about to get her to fall in lust with you at first sight?" Then she turned to Sharon. "No, you Sharon. What did you two talk about when you first met?"

"Literature, art, and travel."

"Things you both like, correct? Was he arrogant, did you argue, and did you have to educate him on things he thought he knew?" Sigrid smiled at Dave as Sharon answered. "Yes, yes, and yes. He tried to convince me his literary hero, Hemingway, wasn't a chauvinist warmonger."

Sigrid looked around the table. "And you Connie and Harvin, and you Audrey and Jake, did you not discuss things you had in common when you first met? Is that not why you connected with each other? Henry and I are researchers, that's what we have in common, so we discussed infectious disease and immunology."

"That's enough grilling. I need a real drink; I'm trading this Champagne in for a Scotch. Anyone else want to hit the bar? Can I bring you something, Sigrid?"

"No, I will go with you." Sigrid stood up as Henry rushed to pull her chair out.

Dave watched them walk away. "Henry is in love. I never thought I would see it, but he is smitten. I just hope she is as smitten as he is."

"She is. She has him hooked, the hook is set, and she has reeled him in." Sharon's eyes were dancing with delight.

"Is that what you did to me?" He leaned toward her.

"Little bit, only you scared me at first, and I wasn't sure I wanted to reel you in, then you started that macho Hemingway BS, and I almost threw you back." She laughed.

"I like her." Audrey said as she watched them.

"So do I," Connie added. "She is head and shoulders above Sherry, literally and figuratively." They all laughed.

"I can tell you one thing; she is smart, and did you see her body? She is an athlete. She's Henry's equal in every way. I like her too, and I can see why Henry fell for her." Dave added.

"She completes us. Henry needed someone for us to be whole. Hot damn, we all got it going on. I am sorry, I don't want to get emotional, but I feel so fortunate. I yearned for nights like this, and friends like you guys, when I was in the service." Jake raised his glass. "Am I glad to be home, with the woman I love, and friends." He was a little choked up as they clinked glasses and drank.

"You know, Jake is right. We are all truly fortunate, and we should be grateful for the kind of lives we have and the friends we have. Happy

New Year, everyone." Harvin raised his glass, and they toasted the New Year. That was the end of the Champagne, so the men joined Henry and Sigrid at the bar.

Dave asked, "Sigrid, you look like an athlete, did you participate in sports at school? Jake and I played American football and Henry was a swimmer."

"Henry, you were a swimmer?" She examined Henry closely.

"He didn't tell you? He still holds some records. Henry, didn't you hold the world record in something at one time, and don't you still hold some American records?"

Henry looked annoyed. "I held the world record in the 200-meter fly very, very briefly, at one meet. I don't follow swimming anymore since I stopped competing." He put his arm around Sigrid. "I would much rather do joint studies on infectious disease and immunology."

"I was involved in sports at university, but I stopped competing to focus on my academics. I was a long jumper and ran some sprints but now I just work out regularly to keep in shape."

"I work out regularly too, and if we ever get to this bar, I'll show you what I do to keep my right arm in shape." Henry pulled her closer.

Sigrid untangled herself from Henry. "Now that the boys are here to keep you company, I will rejoin the girls. Get me a glass of Riesling, please." Henry watched her as she walked back to the table. "I'm going to preempt you, my friend. You can go right down the line with all the things I said to you about Sharon, and right here, right now, I will tell you don't have to say a word. You're right."

"Does she know how wealthy you are?" Dave knew she had to know Henry had money from his car and clothes.

"She knows. When I told her about my trust fund and my family's holdings, she laughed at me and asked if money was all we Americans ever thought about. She accused me of being like all American men, obsessed with money and sex. I couldn't believe a woman got mad at me for telling her I had money. She said my family and I were evil for hoarding money and not sharing it with those in need."

"Did you convince her you weren't obsessed with sex?" Dave laughed.

"No. I can't keep my hands off her. She said, 'You know, Henry, we can have sex anytime; we don't have to have sex all the time.' But I can't help myself. Go ahead and give me a hard time, but you should see the body she has; I mean…, you know what I mean, and she's brilliant. You joked about it, but I get turned on listening to her. When she talks about immunology, it's like she is talking dirty to me. I know you think I am crazy, but she is so damn smart, just listening to her makes me hot for her."

Dave laughed. "Oh man, you got it bad. You is smitten; you is way smitten. You got the fever, man, you got the way high fever. You is burning up with it."

"You is one kettle calling this pot black. You got so much fever I'm surprised you not spontaneously combust." Henry was in love, and his love for Sigrid filled him with a joy he had never experienced before.

Audrey greeted Sigrid when she returned to the table. "You two are an item: it's obvious from across the room."

Sigrid blushed a little. "What does it mean, an item? Does it mean if we are an item, we are lovers?"

Sharon answered. "Little bit. And if Henry is anything like his friend, Dave, it is more than just a little bit."

Sigrid's blush increased. "Maybe he is a little like his friend. We have been together almost constantly since we met, unless of course he is at the hospital. I feel guilty because I have neglected my work to be with him. He is very intense. Are all American men so intense?"

Connie got up. "Come on, girls." They all moved around the table to sit on each side of Sigrid. "Sigrid, he is intense because of you; you make him intense. Normally, Henry is anything but intense."

"Your men are also intense?"

"Sigrid, all men are intense when it comes to being an item."

"I have not had many lovers. I have always been focused on my academics, busy with sports, and now I am engrossed in my research. Then along comes this intense American man and changes everything."

Audrey was sitting on one side of Sigrid. "I think I can speak for all three of us when I say the same thing happened to us. We were all living our lives when along came a man who turned our lives upside down."

The men returned with drinks and were met with a chorus of, "You guys sit over there; we are sitting with our new friend Sigrid." "No boys allowed." "She needs to be protected from intense American men."

The orchestra began to play, and Sharon led Dave to the dance floor. She swirled into the dance; light and graceful in his arms. She floated joyfully on the music, happy, and as carefree as a child. He put his lips near her ear and whispered, "You look wonderful tonight. I'll never forget the way you look tonight." They danced until the band took a break, and as they walked back to the table, he noticed Sigrid watching them. Despite the cold blueness of their color, her eyes conveyed warmth and understanding.

During the break, he learned she had progressed through school at an accelerated pace, earning her PhD in her early twenties. She was younger than the rest of them but seemed more mature than any of them. She was a scientist, but she was well rounded, well read, and had backpacked through most of Europe. Jake was right, she completed them. They were all bright with a sense of purpose to their lives. They fit together as a group. Dave thought how privileged they were compared to the patients he saw at University Hospital. Henry was right too, because of their privilege, they were obligated to make some sort of contribution. And Mama was right: they were blessed, and they should never forget to share their blessings.

Henry talked to Dave at the bar during the break. "Sigrid is only here for six months. She will finish her research project and go back to Denmark. She has a place on the university staff there so she's planning to return to teach and continue her research. I don't know what to do. She has her career, I have mine, and the Atlantic Ocean is between us. I can't give up my dream, and I can't ask her to give up hers."

"Find a way to make it work, Henry. I could never be happy without Sharon, and I will do whatever it takes to keep her in my life. Do whatever it takes to keep Sigrid in your life."

"You do mess with a man's head with all your romantic notions, Dave. It scares the hell out of me to think about changing my whole life for a woman. My logical mind rejects emotional decisions like that."

"You're not changing your life for a woman, you're changing it for love, and there is no decision to be made, emotional or otherwise. You choose love or live with regret for the rest of your life. Choose love, Henry."

When they came back to the table, Sigrid looked at them with an amused expression. "I saw you two talking. Should I be worried?"

"No, there is nothing to worry about. I can see that now." Henry sat down.

Midnight came, Dave and Sharon kissed, toasted the New Year with Champagne, sang Auld Lang Syne, and danced until the party ended. Their room had a king-size bed and a floor-to-ceiling window overlooking the city. Once they were in the room, Sharon took her bag and went to the bathroom.

Dave was in bed when she opened the bathroom door and stood in it in a sheer negligee with the light behind. He was out of bed immediately, but she ignored him, walked to the floor-to-ceiling window, pulled the curtain back, and stood in the window with her arms stretched out touching each side of the opening. Their room wasn't very high and if anyone on the street had looked up, they would have seen a beautiful woman standing in the window gazing out at the city, but it was late, so no one saw the apparition in the window.

Dave walked up behind her, put his arms around her, and she put her head over so he could nuzzle her neck, but she didn't move or turn from the window. All the buildings had left their lights on for New Year's Eve, so the city was aglow with white and colored lights. Looking out the window was like looking into a giant kaleidoscope of colors and shapes.

"Caroline will marry Ron and move to New York, because that is where he needs to be for his career. Audrey will marry Jake, he will get promoted, and they will move to a different base. Connie and Harvin are going to California after they marry. Who knows what will become of Sigrid and Henry? They are from two different countries, thousands of miles apart. We will all go our separate ways and never be together again like we are now. Promise me we will stay in touch with our friends no matter where they are." She turned in his arms. The feel of her body through the negligee was too much for him. He scooped her up and carried her to the bed.

Dave woke up with Sharon on top of him, her hair down around his face, and he could smell Chanel and her body lotion. "You were ready, so I started without you." She laughed. "Now it's my turn to take care of you." And she did. They made love with the morning light streaming through the big window bathing them in its warmth.

Afterwards, they stayed in bed enjoying the feel of their bodies pressed against each other until Sharon sat up. "Let's try out the tub." She went to the bathroom to fill the tub. The negligee was long gone, and Dave watched her walk to and from the bathroom. *Her body really is perfect, she really is beautiful, and I'm really going to spend my life with her.* She came to the bed and pulled him up by the hand. "Come on, this tub is great, you would think you had never seen me naked before. Stop ogling me and let's have fun in the tub. You wanted to go skinny dipping: well, let's go skinny dipping."

He grabbed her and pulled her down on the bed. "I want to live here. We can live here and never get dressed or leave this room. We'll make love all the time and order room service when we get hungry." She wiggled free and ran to the bathroom. "Come on, the tub is about to run over." They bathed each other and used the hand attachment to wash their hair. After they got out and toweled off, they put their robes on, and Sharon started looking for her negligee. "Where is my negligee? I wasn't in complete control of my faculties when it came off, so I have no idea how it got off, or where it is." She found the negligee buried in the sheets. "Do you know when check-out is? We could order room service and have breakfast in bed." Dave called the front desk, and they told him check-out was at noon, and transferred him to room service to order breakfast.

She walked back to stand in the window looking out again. "What a wonderful way to start the new year. When last year started, I could never have imagined it would end the way it did last night, and in my wildest dreams I couldn't have conceived of this year starting the way it did this morning. I want to spend every New Year's Eve in a hotel."

She came back and lay across the bed on her stomach with her chin in her hands. "I wonder where being with you will take me from here and how much more it will change my life." She rolled onto her back. "It has already been a wild ride far beyond my comfort zone. How much more is there to experience? Sigrid was right about men like you. You're intense, the ride is scary, and feels out of control sometimes, but it is also wonderful, and I never want it to end. How dull and unfulfilled my life would have been if I hadn't met you and been exposed to your inquisitive mind, your need to know, your need to experience, to participate and be involved: your need to live life to the fullest. Like I told you when I met you, it's what's above your shoulders, not what is below the waist that's important to me. But you taught me about what is below your waist too, Jesus, have you ever taught me about that, and last night was an incredible lesson."

Chapter 10

OB/GYN

The shifts in the OB/GYN ER were twenty-four hours on, and twenty-four hours off. There were no teams and Dave worked with different students, interns, and residents depending on their schedules. All pregnant patients went upstairs to L and D, and most of the cases he saw were boring and repetitive; consisting of STDs, vaginitis, pelvic inflammatory disease, excessive vaginal bleeding or dysfunctional bleeding, abdominal pain, painful intercourse, abscesses, and UTIs.

A lot of the patients were from the Afro-American and the Latino neighborhoods where they live in poverty. White flight from the city to the gated communities of the suburbs had created and perpetuated an economic form of segregation. In the remaining city neighborhoods and the surrounding underprivileged rural areas, it was as if the conditions of the Great Depression that Steinbeck described in The Grapes of Wrath still exist. Both Dickens and Steinbeck emphasized the corrosive effects of poverty on a society, the damage it did, and how it infected the whole culture with an underlying toxic darkness, yet Dave confronted Dickens' children of mankind, Ignorance and Want, every day in University Hospital's ED. He knew a lot of it was tied to racism, but some of the impoverished were white, so it wasn't all be based on race. Lack of education and opportunity were factors that crossed the color line.

The inhabitants of the rundown, crime ridden, drug infested ethnic neighborhoods in the city and of the poor rural areas that surround it live in pockets of poverty that resemble third world countries embedded in the richest nation in the world. Many of the neighborhoods and outlying rural areas are like foreign territories where the residents don't speak

English, or they communicate in a dialect indigenous to their culture or their particular neighborhood. Others have no home, but live on the streets, in tents under the overpasses, or in the wooded areas of the city. The impoverished provide a plethora of patients for University Hospital.

The elderly residents of these neighborhoods and rural areas are often neglected. One of the worst cases of neglect he dealt with was an elderly Black woman who presented with a "sore on her breast". A kindly neighbor woman brought her to the ED by bus. She was thin and bent with snow white hair. Her worn oversized dress was pressed, and clean as were her battered shoes. She carried a large, ragged straw bag, and wore wire rimmed glasses set low on her nose. Despite her appearance, she had a certain dignity and pride in her bearing. She was very reluctant to show Dave the "sore on her breast" and was genuinely embarrassed at having to expose herself. The "sore" on her right breast was a fungating carcinoma with superficial necrosis that had destroyed her entire breast. Her name was Rosalie. She was bright, well-spoken, and educated with an obvious sense of decorum. It wasn't terribly busy, so Dave sat in the exam area with her and kept her company to help elevate her fears while they waited for the on-call Surgery team. She told him she was a schoolteacher and she had worked until she couldn't make it to and from the rural school where she taught any more. Her family had simply melted away; moved, married, died, or disappeared leaving her alone after she stopped teaching. She took in washing and ironing from neighbors and kept chickens to sell the eggs to support herself. When the Surgery team took her away, she smiled pleasantly at Dave and thanked him for being so kind. As he watched her being wheeled down the hall on the gurney, a sadness seeped into his heart; a type of grief or mourning for the plight of humanity in all its suffering forms including this fine old woman struggling through the twilight of her life all alone.

The worst case of racism Dave encountered during his internship involved a poor white couple who lived in the same circumstances as their Black neighbors. There was an Afro-American RN on the three-to-eleven shift who warmed up to Dave after she watched him with the woman with breast cancer. They both enjoyed music and were discussing the Blue's influence on Jazz one night when his student approached him. "There is a man who won't let me see his wife. He said he doesn't want a short-coat doctor; he wants a long-coat doctor." Many of the patients who frequented University Hospital knew students wore short coats, and MDs wore long lab coats. "Let's go Ella. We'll give him an RD, real doctor, and an RN, real nurse."

When Dave pulled the curtain back, the husband yelled at him. "Get that nigger out of here. She's not touching my wife, and neither are you. You're not a doctor; not with that hair." The man's breath smelled of stale beer, his fingernails were ragged and dirty, his skin was pallid, his eyes were bloodshot, and his clothes were grimy. "She is a registered nurse, and I am an MD, but if you don't want us, I will put your chart back, and you can wait until a white nurse and a doctor with short hair are available."

"We been waiting long enough; you get someone right now!" Dave realized the man was drunk. He backed out of the exam area and turned to Ella. "Get security." When the Black security guards showed up, the husband went off on them with the same racist rhetoric, but they got control of him quickly, and escorted him out of the ED as quietly as possible.

Dave and Ella walked back to the doctor's station together. "I am sorry. You didn't deserve that."

"Do you think that is the first time something like that has happened to me? I deal with it all the time."

"You're an excellent nurse. Why don't you leave and go where things like this don't happen? I am applying to programs in California for my residency. Why don't you move out of the South?"

She shook her head. "Do you think you can move away from racism and make a geographical solution to the problem? I am a single mom with kids, and I take care of my mother who worked two jobs to put me through nursing school. She cleaned white people's toilets as a maid for a white family during the day and worked for a janitorial service cleaning white people's toilet in a high-rise office building at night. What am I supposed to do, move someplace without a job or any means of support with my mother and kids? This is my home. I was born and raised here. What makes you think it's any better in California, the promised land, do you really believe in that fantasy? You can't make a geographic solution to your problems. You're a dreamer Dave, but it's a pleasure working with someone like you. Someone who can hang with John Lee Hooker." She laughed.

Ella loaned Dave some of her vinyl records to play at his apartment with Sharon, and when he told her about Ellen, she responded. "You and I can never know what she deals with every day or what her life has been like. God, she must have a lot of courage. Please thank her for the music and let her know how much I enjoyed the records, but also tell her from one woman to another how much I admire her courage." When he told Ella what Sharon had said about her courage, she looked surprised, then said. "Tell my white sister she is welcome."

But it was the rape cases that bothered Dave the most. In all rape cases the victims have to be examined for injury and a rape kit used to collect evidence. The victims of violent rapes often ended up in the Surgery ER or in the Trauma Unit, but a GYN exam still must be performed, and a rape kit used to collect evidence. The violent gang rapes and rapes were the rapists tortured or mutilated their victims left the women not only psychologically scared, but physically injured and often permanently disfigured. There were also the girls and women who the rapist murdered in the process of raping them. They were handled by the coroner's office when they were found: if they were found.

It angered Dave to see what the rapists did to the girls and women they raped, but his disgust increased when he saw how rape victims were treated by the system. If the victim knew their assailant, it was a case of "he said - she said." In cases where the victim didn't know their assailant, the man still said the sex was consensual. Even in cases of gang rape, the men said the woman or girl wanted to pull a train and it was her word against theirs. The rapists always said it was consensual no matter what the circumstances.

A young college girl was brought in by her roommate after she was raped by another student she had seen on the campus multiple times. He caught her in an isolated area at night and raped her. If she made a sound, he hit her, if she did not do what he told her to do, he hit her, if she was not fully cooperative, he hit her. Not only was she savagely beaten about the face, but she also had vaginal trauma indicating forceful penetration.

She told her story to the investigating officer, and Dave reported what he found on her exam, including the extent of her facial and vaginal injuries. She said there were pictures of all the students on file in the dean's office and she was sure she could identify her assailant. The officer only asked one question: were there any witnesses? When she said no, he told her even if she identified his picture, it was his word against hers. He suggested she dressed too provocatively, and maybe she was raped because she enticed her assailant with her appearance.

That was too much for Dave. He got in the officer's face and went Texas Tom on him. "You are worthless as a police officer, and you are more worthless as a human being. Get out of my ER and send someone in here to help this girl who is not a flaming asshole."

The second officer told him there were hundreds of rape kits sitting on a shelf in the evidence room because the DA's office would not prosecute a case they could not win, and it was hard to win a: he said, she said case. The victim reports a rape, but the rapist states it was consensual sex and with no witnesses, it is his word against hers, so the detectives saw no reason to waste time investigating the rape or having the kit processed if the DA was not going to prosecute. Dave pointed out the facial and vaginal injuries, the history of stalking, and the girl's emotional state. The officer said it was still his word against hers and even if there was DNA evidence in the rape kit to link him to the rape, he would say it was consensual. He added it took a unanimous vote to convict, and the men on a jury tended to side with the male assailant.

The second officer made out a report, but he told the girl the same things he told Dave. The poor girl felt abandoned. She cried uncontrollably and all Dave could do was call Psych to see her. He realized these poor women and girls were not only traumatized by the rape; they were further emotionally damaged by their treatment from the justice system. The rape kit exam was bad enough, but to be made to think the rape was their fault, or that nothing could or would be done about it crushed them completely.

Dave was becoming ashamed of his gender: the rape, the guy at the pool, the guys in the hotel, and all other men who hit on Sharon every day. His disdain for men who rape, men who thought they could buy any woman they wanted like a commodity, and men who hit on women pushing their unwanted advances on them escalated into a concern for Sharon's safety. He bought a Taser and a can of pepper spray for Sharon to carry and asked her to have an airport security guard walk her to and from her car at night. She protested, but he told her it was not up for discussion.

She tried to get Henry to do an intervention to calm him down, but that resulted in Henry buying Sigrid a small handgun to carry in her purse when he found out a rape occurred on the university campus where she was doing her research. He demanded she not work late, leave the campus before dark, and carry the gun. When she refused the gun, and accused him of being a crazy American cowboy, he got her a Taser. It spilled over to Harvin from Henry and Connie found herself with a Taser, Harvin walking her to her car when he was at the hospital, and a security guard when he was not available. The women got together and tried to confront their men, but they were argued down by the statistics Dave found on sexual assaults in a study done by a women's research group.

"I know the three of you think you're liberated, but you still have a long way to go. This study shows almost all women experience a sexual assault at least once during their life. We aren't going to take any risk where you're concerned. These precautions are prudent and necessary. Students, nurses, and flight attendants are particularly vulnerable because of late shifts, late trips, or late-night study habits." Dave was adamant, as were Henry and Harvin.

He said goodbye to Ella on his last shift in the GYN ED. The last day of his ED rotations had to be a day off to keep him from working straight through, but having the first day off on the next rotation had been just luck: his luck held and his first day in Labor and Delivery was an off day.

The New York Metropolitan Ballet Company was touring, and they were performing at the Civic Center in the city, so he bought tickets for his night off. A ballet always draws attractive people dressed to be seen, and they stood in the lobby sipping Champagne, watching the couples arrive until the first bell rang. "I had forgotten how glamorous the ballet was. When I went to college, I walked away from it and buried myself in my studies, but I want to be a part of it again. Not to dance of course, but to be a part of it, like tonight. I am so glad we came." Sharon continued to find herself through Dave. The other men she dated, including Bar, would have scoffed at going to a ballet, but he was excited when he told he had tickets. She was sure he wanted to go, but she was also sure he wanted to take her to something she had loved and lost in the hope she would find it again. She did.

The ballet was excellent, and it was all very sensual in a subtle romantic way emphasizing the human form in a series of stylized dance movements. After it ended, they walked to a small café near the theater for a glass of wine and a light supper. The café was a romantic rendezvous for lovers from the theater sharing one last moment with the world before retiring to consummate their love. Their lovemaking that night was like the ballet; romantic and filled with subtle passion.

She was already up when he woke up. "What are we going to do today?"

"I'm going to call Henry and see if they want to come over and hang out. We can order a couple of pizzas for dinner."

Dave called Henry as soon as he was dressed. "Are you up. If you are, I can call back later."

Henry answered, "Very funny." Dave asked if he and Sigrid wanted to get together and hang out. "Wait, I'll ask Sigrid. She's mad at me because I kept her from going to the lab this morning. That thing you asked about, you know, being up." Henry asked Sigrid if she wanted to take the rest of the day off since it was nearly half over and hang out with Sharon and Dave. "She said she will hang out with you guys but not with me because I'm a bad man who prevents the advancement of science to gratify my carnal desires. I swear to God that's what she said. Jesus, she just hit me. Give us some time to clean up and for me to get treatment for my bruises. She hit me again. Sigrid, stop hitting me. She said I deserve it for making her neglect her research, then talking to you about why. Who knew Danes were so abusive? See you later."

Sigrid and Henry arrived that afternoon with four bottles of wine. Henry was dressed like Henry was always dressed, only he had on a down jacket. Sigrid was in jeans, a white ski sweater with dark blue patterns woven into it that accentuated her eyes, a blue woolen scarf, a blue ski jacket, and calf-high, fur-lined, lace-up boots with heels.

Dave ushered them in and took the bottles of wine. "Jesus, Henry, we're ordering pizza. Are you sure you want to drink these with pizza?" He had brought two bottles of Grand Cru Bordeaux and two bottles of French Burgundy.

"Open the Burgundy first and we'll drink the Bordeaux later." The beanbags were oversized so Henry and Sigrid could easily fit in one together, but Sigrid made Henry sit on the floor in front of her. "I needed to go to the lab this morning, but he wanted to play, so he overrode my wishes and we played, but his play time with me is over. I am here to visit with you. He can sit on the floor and play with himself now."

Dave came out of the kitchen with two glasses of wine. "He can't play with himself in front of me." He handed one glass to Sigrid and the other to Sharon who sat down in the other bean bag.

"What kind of a guy takes advantage of a poor foreign girl's lack of understanding of the language to joke about his friend?" Henry situated himself on the floor.

He came back with two more glasses of wine and handed one to Henry. "Sigrid's English is better than mine. She is the one who made the joke. I just delivered the punch line." He raised his glass. "Skol." They all repeated "Skol" and took a sip of wine. He started the music with the volume low enough to allow them to talk and went to sit with Sharon. "If Henry has to sit on the floor, so do you."

"What did I do?"

"You are a sexual harasser just like Henry. You two harassers can sit together on the floor and play with each other now." Sharon laughed at her own joke.

"Very funny." Dave sat down on the floor with Henry.

The music was good, the wine was excellent, and eventually Henry slid in beside Sigrid and Dave joined Sharon. The hospital and all it represented was on another planet a million light years away as they talked, listened to music, and drank French wine.

As afternoon evolved into evening, Sigrid sat up. "It is so good to relax with wine, music, and friends. It reminds me of home. In Denmark, the days are so short in winter, and it is so cold, we spend a lot of time like this, visiting and talking. Henry must do something all of the time. We go out to dinner, we go here, we go there, we go somewhere and do something all the time, and if we are not going and doing, we are an item." Sigrid laid back in Henry's arms. "I wonder why we can't have more time like this."

"It is because he needs to be distracted. Dave is the same way, intense. That's what you said. They're intense. I know exactly how you feel because I feel the same way. I even thought there might be something wrong with us because we did it too much."

"Yes!"

"Then I realized the beauty of our lovemaking replaces the ugliness he is exposed to at the hospital, so I embraced it, and boy does he need a lot of embracing."

Sigrid sat up and looked at Henry. "Is that why you must be so busy all the time? You need distracting."

In all the years Dave had known Henry, he had never seen him vulnerable, speechless, or emotional, but his face softened considerably as he put his arms around Sigrid and pulled her to him without saying anything.

"OK, I keep you distracted, but can we do this too? I would like an afternoon like this from time to time."

Henry got up to open another bottle of wine. "You're right, Sigrid. I had forgotten how good it is to simply hang out with friends, talk, listen to music, and share a bottle of wine." He came back and filled their glasses and lifted his glass. "Skol, brother, we definitely have to do this more often."

"Skol, brother." Dave had forgotten how much he depended on Henry.

Sharon took a sip of the wine. "We can do this as often as you like, Henry, if you bring the wine."

Henry told them he had located a flat in an apartment building in the city closer to the hospital. Sigrid added, "I am glad he is moving, because Mike keeps walking in on me when I am in the shower. He listens for the shower, then walks in the bathroom like he did not know I was there. I have been to nude beaches in Europe, so I am used to being seen without clothes, but this is different. I want to cover up when he looks at me. It is not like at the beach in France where you feel admired when men look at you."

They spent the rest of the evening drinking wine, listening to music, and talking wrapped in a warm blanket of friendship.

On Dave's first shift in L and D he delivered Big John, or actually he fumbled him into the world. His mother named him John because all the nurses called him Big John from the minute he entered the world. She was a small woman whose abdomen was so large it looked as if her skin was going to split when she presented to L and D. At first, he was sure she had full-term twins, but her exam and ultrasound showed only one fetus and one heartbeat. He checked her for diabetes since the baby was so large, but her labs were normal. It was her first baby, so she was exhausted from a long, hard labor when he finally took her to the delivery room.

Newborn babies are slippery. When Big John crowned, Dave cut a large episiotomy, but his head was so big it tore everything anyway, and he just kept coming, shoulders, body, all of him, all at once. Dave tried desperately to get a grip on him, but he was just too big, too heavy, too slippery, and coming too fast. Dave kept grabbing at him as he slid toward the kick bucket at the foot of the delivery table and finally fumbling him into the bucket as if he were trying to help him into it. The second John hit the kick bucket, he let out a scream. He was huge, and the contents of the kick bucket made him even more slippery, so Dave could not get him out of the bucket as he continued to scream at the top of his lungs.

"Where's my baby?" the mother asked.

"He is right here. We'll have him with you in a minute." But Dave could not get a grip on him because both John and Dave's hands were even more slippery from the contents of the kick bucket, so John remained in the kick bucket screaming. The nurse came to his aid and together, they were finally able to get John over to the warmer. He never stopped screaming the whole time.

"Where's my baby? Is he all right?" the mother kept asking.

"He's fine. He's a big healthy boy. We just need to clean him up, weigh him, and get his vitals."

"What Apgar?" the nurse asked.

"Twelve!" Dave answered. John weighed fourteen pounds, twice the weight of a normal baby, and it took Dave an hour to repair the damage he did to his mother's bottom. He immediately became the nurses' favorite, and they all called him Big John, so the mother had no choice but to name him John.

The interns and students did all the normal deliveries with the residents only intervening when the mother needed a C-section or there was a problem with the presentation, like a breach. At first, Dave assisted the resident when a baby got in trouble with a declining heart rate and needed an emergency C-section, then after he had done a few with the resident assisting him, he began to do them with a student assisting him. An emergency C-section was a race to get the baby out before it suffered any damage from hypoxia and that aroused his competitive nature. He enjoyed doing C-sections like he had enjoyed doing procedures in general surgery.

But there were also problems in L and D: mothers with Preëclampsia or Eclampsia (toxemia), diabetic mothers, and mothers with drug or alcohol addiction. Unfortunately, the specter of poverty and all it brought with it loomed over the delivery room too. But he liked delivering babies, and there were their proud, happy, loving mothers, so he slogged through poverty, lack of education, heart ache, tragedy, and disasters doing what he could to help.

Death occurred in L and D, but death in L and D, where it was supposed to be about new life, whether it was the death of the mother or the child, was particularly unsettling. On one of his shifts, Trauma One notified Land D they had a mother near term who had suffered a lethal head injury in an MVA. When Dave and the resident got to Trauma 1, they found the mother on life support, but the baby had a good strong heartbeat, so they did a C-section and delivered a healthy baby boy. The resident went back to L and D and left him to deal with the father.

Dave and the trauma resident took the husband, and now new father, to a side room in the ED waiting area to have him sign papers to remove his wife from life support, and to tell him he could see his newborn son in the nursery. In one fleeting moment he had to deal with the dichotomy of losing his wife and gaining a son. One is the most wonderful thing that can happen to a man, and the other is the worst thing that could happen to a husband. Dave would never forget the expressions on the man's face or the mixed emotions he exhibited at hearing both things simultaneously. The whole incident left him with the impression that life was far too complicated for him to comprehend. He concluded: life is what it is, so acknowledge it, and move on, because there is nothing else you can do. He acquired one more tool to help him deal with the tragedies he was exposed to: another type of shovel to use to bury them in his graveyard of the unthinkable and unacceptable.

Valentine's Day came and went with him working a shift in L and D and Sharon flying. He sent her flowers and a card she found in her room when she got back from her trip, and she took him a box of candy with a card the next day. But he would always remember that Valentine's Day because of a young woman and her baby girl. She was seventeen. The young man with her was about the same age, and neither spoke English. The interpreter told Dave they left Mexico because of the stigma of an unmarried pregnancy and the desire for a better life for themselves and their child. She had walked a thousand miles from Mexico, and they only stopped because she went into labor.

Married or not, it was obvious they were very much in love. The interpreter had to pull them apart to get her into a room and into a bed. Her labor was going fine until the monitor sounded an alarm as the heart rate of the baby dropped drastically. Dave did not hesitate. He called for the nurse and started wheeling the bed to the OR, yelling orders as he went. The young man was left dumbfounded and speechless as watched the chaos.

She was moved to the OR table screaming in fear because she did not understand what was happening. Anesthesia arrived and a quick prep was done on her abdomen. Dave had the baby out in no time. The infant girl was blue because the cord was wrapped around her neck, and it was obstructed. As the baby moved down the birth canal during labor, the cord tightened and occluded. If he had not been in the room when the cord occluded, the baby could have been still born. If he had not gotten the baby out so quickly, she could have had brain damage. But because he was examining her when it happened and acted quickly, he was able to present the young man with a healthy baby girl. He wept as he held his new daughter for the first time, and Dave felt a surge of emotion. He had saved a newborn life and given a young couple a future. A future where they hoped to give their infant girl a better life. He experienced a feeling of indescribable exhilaration as he watched the father with his baby daughter.

He walked out of the hospital the next morning, looked up at the icy blue sky, felt the crisp chill of the beginning of a new winter's day, and realized he had done something wonderful. He had made a difference, not just in the baby girl's and her parents' lives, but in the overall scheme of things. In a tiny, minute way he had changed the course of the universe by changing the course of the baby's future, and more importantly he had defeated death. He had not only prevented suffering and disability: he had prevented a death. As he stood there looking up at the sky and enjoying the freshness of the new day, it all came together for him. *I get it, Sheffield. I finally get it.*

On the day after Dave's last shift in L and D, Henry invited everyone over for a get-together at his new apartment. He was up, showered, shaved, and dressed when Sharon arrived. It was the end of February and cold, so she had on jeans, boots, and a ski sweater with a puffy down jacket over the sweater.

When they arrived, Dave looked around the flat and pulled Henry aside. "She is not a bird or a fish, Henry."

"Biology is biology, Dave. I need keep her here until I finish my training." In certain species of birds and fish, the male builds a nest to attract a female. The better the male is at building the nest, and the better the nest is, the better the male chances are of attracting the female of his choice. Ever the biologist, Henry had built a nest to attract the female of his choice and keep her from returning to Denmark.

The flat was big, and Henry had spared no expense in decorating it in a purely Scandinavian style. It had two bedrooms, two baths, a formal dining room, a large living room, and a spacious kitchen with a breakfast area. The furniture was all light wood with glass, the lamps and fixtures were tasteful, and original prints by Chagall and Matisse adorned the walls. Dave looked at the prints. "Who are her favorite artists? Let me guess, could they be Chagall and Matisse?"

"I love her, Dave. You are the one who told me not to lose her. I want to spend my life with her, but she doesn't like it here, and wants to go back to Denmark. I need to stay here long enough to finish my residency and do a fellowship, then I will go to Europe with her. I can work for the International CDC. We could even work together and become a research team. I don't want to take her away from her family and her country, but I want to finish my training."

"Your family can donate to the program and extend the research grant for her project. You can pay for her to fly home first class and see her family as often as she wants. Tell her that. Tell her you want to spend your life with her, and you want the two of you to become a research team. Woo her, Henry. Woo her with double-blind studies like we joked about. You built her a nest, now woo her."

While Dave and Henry were talking, Sigrid sought out Sharon and found her talking to Connie. "Sigrid, I love your style. Are all your clothes from Europe?" Sigrid was dressed in a light blue cocktail dress that matched her eyes with a darker blue silk scarf and heels that matched the scarf. "You look like a Nordic princess."

"Thank you, Sharon. I brought everything with me from Denmark. Henry keeps trying to buy me clothes, jewelry, other things but that makes me uncomfortable and look at this flat. I want to talk to you about Henry and this flat."

"Obviously, it's a shrine to you. So, what's the problem?" Sharon laughed.

"I do not want to stay in America. I want to finish my project and go home. I miss my mother, father, brother, and all my friends in Denmark. I do not like it here. I do not like the culture and the problems in your society. People are so much happier in Denmark. Things are so much more relaxed and easier there. I know he decorated this flat to entice me to live with him, but I want to go home."

"If you love Henry, you should be with him, but you should be happy too. Love should fulfill your happiness, not take it away from you." Connie wondered how hard it would be to maintain a long-distance relationship across the Atlantic Ocean.

Sigrid looked at Sharon. "What should I do about moving in with Henry? My research grant pays for room and board, a car, and expenses until May. It would be a waste if I moved in with him, and I would feel as if I were giving up my freedom. That is another problem. Henry's money and what it can buy, like this flat. I am afraid of his money, the control it has over him, and the control it could have over me. I do not want to have my life dominated by money. I would be yielding to this lavish apartment, letting it and Henry's money control me, if I move in with him." Sigrid had always been conflicted by her relationship with Henry.

"Keep your place and stay there when Henry is at the hospital. Move some stuff here and stay here when you can be with Henry. That is what we do. Sharon stays at Dave's when they can be together, then she stays at her house when Dave is at the hospital. I do the same thing; except we stay at my place when Harvin and I can be together because I live alone. That's a simple solution and it works; we can vouch for that." Connie felt satisfied that she had helped solve at least one of Sigrid's problems.

The party broke up around six and everyone left Henry and Sigrid to work out their impending problem of an unhappy Sigrid, or a very long-distance romance. After Sharon told Dave about her conversation with Sigrid, he thought about the wealthy men trying to buy Sharon in the hotel.

This was the first time Henry had dated someone not of his socio-economic class and now Dave understood why. He concluded Henry and Sigrid were facing bigger obstacles than the Atlantic Ocean, and he wondered if any amount of love could overcome the problems that were forced on them by their circumstances.

Dave rotated to the OB/GYN wards. Their applications were in, and they planned their vacation for May. The OB/GYN wards' schedule was like the Surgery wards schedule with every third day on call and the day after call off once rounds were made. Elective surgeries were in the morning and clinic was in the afternoon of the day before call. His surgery and clinic day was a long, hard twelve-hours, but he had the afternoon and night after call off.

Pregnant women admitted for control of their diabetes, blood pressure, or any other complication of pregnancy were admitted by the residents. He only admitted gynecological disorders.

In clinic he treated sexually transmitted diseases; everything from pubic lice, commonly known as crabs, to gonorrhea, and even one case of syphilis. He also saw women from higher socioeconomic levels. These women came to the University Hospital GYN Clinic because they thought or knew they had something and were embarrassed to go to their private doctors. They did not want an STD noted in their regular medical record. He also treated working girls, lower-class street prostitutes, but there were some high-end escorts who came to be tested on a regular basis.

The cancer cases were troubling because cervical cancer, uterine cancer, and breast cancer were curable if they were diagnosed and treated early. HPV vaccinations, universal cervical and uterine cancer screening with a PAP smear and pelvic exam, along with mammograms and breast exams could save lives. The uninsured, about thirty percent of the population, had no access to these simple screening tests. The patients at University Hospital received free screening, but they were a fraction of the underserved women in the community.

He could not understand why there was not government funding for universal cancer screening for women. He felt that not providing free vaccinations and screening was not only negligent but was criminal. Withholding lifesaving women's healthcare was murder on a grand sociological scale by the politicians who blocked any attempts to institute government funded health programs.

Dave hated politicians who wrapped themselves in the flag and presented themselves as devout Christians but voted against any healthcare measures. They voted for huge sums for the military to fund unwinnable, endless wars, but they refused to vote for any funds for healthcare and screamed *"SOCIALISM,"* at the top of their lungs any time a healthcare bill came to the floor. They voted to kill on a mass scale but refused to vote to save lives on any scale. They presented themselves as God's servants, doing God's work, for patriotic reasons, protecting and promoting the American way of life by supported the gun lobby and NRA but would not support lifesaving public health measures. The word "hypocrite" was far too mild for them.

Dave's believed routine, accurate screening tests, vaccinations, and anything having to do with public health should be paid for by the public. It was the public's health; therefore, it should be paid for by the public and available to all the public. During his trip to Europe, the people he met questioned him about healthcare in the US once they found out he was a medical student. They were incredulous and could not believe the US didn't provide health care for all its citizens. The idea that some people and politicians have that if you can't afford care, you don't get care, was repugnant to them. Once he confirmed that some individuals did actually die because they could not afford the treatment they needed, they asked him questions that resonated with him. "What kind of person equates money to a human being's life?" "What is the value of a human life and what type of scale do you use to measure that value?" The idea that who lives and who dies is based on what they can afford was overwhelming to them. "What kind of person, culture, or society promotes such an approach?"

He also saw cases of domestic violence in the Gyn clinic. Most domestic abuse is never reported, and the women suffer the beatings in silence because they are afraid of their abuser. The cases of domestic violence he saw in the Surgery ER presented injuries that needed medical attention. The cases in the Gyn clinic presented with gynecological problems that interfered with or prevented sex. The injuries due to domestic abuse were discovered when the patient was examined, but it was the gynecological problem that brought them to the clinic, and it was the gynecological problem that instigated the abuse that caused injuries.

He saw a working girl with vaginitis. During his exam, Dave discovered bruises on her body that were covered by her clothing. When Dave asked her about the bruising, she became frightened and told him she fell down the stairs. She had been beaten with something like a belt by her pimp because she could not work with vaginitis. She begged Dave not to say anything about it because her pimp took care of her and protected her. She needed him.

A young woman came in because she had trichomoniasis, a sexually transmitted disease. When Dave looked closely at her face, he saw bruises that were hidden by makeup. She contracted the STD from casual sex with someone other than her boyfriend, and the boyfriend beat her with his fist when he contracted it from her. She told Dave she was fine, the beating was her fault, she deserved it for cheating on her boyfriend, and to please let it go.

There was also an undercurrent in the male dominated OB/GYN Department that made him uneasy. It was a subtle attitude that permeated the house staff's interactions with the patients. He had not encountered anything like it in Surgery or Medicine. There were women attendings and women on the OB/GYN house staff, but he did not have an opportunity to work with any of them, so he did not know if they were tainted by it too, but he doubted it. He thought it was a gender-related, unstated belief that women are inferior and could be dealt with in the offhanded dominant way by the males.

He developed a deeper understanding of the courage and strength of women on his OB/GYN rotation. He had seen the strength it took to be a mother from the terminal cancer patient protecting her children from foster care. But it was the entire process of bringing a child into the world that crystallized how strong and courageous women are. A woman's courage reminded him of Melville's description of Starbuck's courage in Moby Dick. It was a commodity, a staple, a solid dependable resource always there when needed.

The courage a woman displays is often motivated by her need to nurture. She carries another human being in her body, goes through the risk and pain of expelling that human being, then nurtures and cares for it until it matures. The strength and courage it took to be a woman was only exceeded by the strength and courage it took to be a mother.

It pained him to think about what Sharon went through every day at work and the strength she had to have to ward off the unwanted attention and advances, deal with the sexual harassment, and keep things from getting out of control. She had to walk a fine line and not create a problem through her rejections, do a good job, and still protect herself. It was hard to be a woman because you were undervalued and over judged. It was harder to be an attractive woman because you were hit on, and she had to deal with the situation in a way that prevented the rejection from escalating into something ugly. Then there was Ella, the Black RN in the ER who had to have even more strength and courage to deal with not only being a woman, but also with being a Black woman and a single mother.

Dave had mixed feelings about his OB/GYN rotation, but he had acquired a deeper understanding of the fundamental truths about the complexity of human existence and how women dealt with those complexities. He was in a good mood on his last day on call, because April brought the change to Pedi, residency offers, and his last three-month rotation.

Chapter 11

Pediatrics

Sheffield told Henry and Mike they could continue at University Hospital for their residency, but he did not talk to Dave, so he had to wait to hear from the USC program at LA County Hospital, or the UCLA program at UCLA Medical Center. He was not asked to interview with Stanford or UCSF.

The Pedi wards were like the Medicine wards. He was on call every third day with the afternoon clinic on the day before and the day after call. There was an attending who met with the house staff and students after morning rounds during the week, a supervising resident over the interns, and the Chief of Pediatrics held Grand Rounds on Saturday at noon.

The Pedi staff from the attendings down to the nurse's aides were kind, gentle, caring people and he found more women house staff in the Pedi department. His supervising resident was a smart, knowledgeable woman with a cheerful disposition and a warm personality.

His service was small, but the children were sick with a variety of ailments. Dealing with sick children was hard, but at least he didn't have to care for the children with cancer. They were on the oncology service. He respected all oncologists, but pediatric oncologists were a breed apart. Being an oncologist is one of the toughest jobs in medicine, but being a pediatric oncologist requires dedication, commitment, and a special kind of empathy beyond the capacity of most physicians. To face every day knowing many of your patients are going to die and continue to fight for their lives was a challenge, but to do it with children was beyond anything he could imagine.

If he was awed by oncologists, he saw oncology nurses as saints. Oncology nurses in general are special people, but Pedi oncology nurses are the most dedicated, caring, resilient women he encountered during his internship. A lot of the Pedi oncology nurses are young. He asked the charge nurse why? She told him most of them burn out after about five years and move on to another service. But a few like herself could not walk away knowing how much the children and their families needed them. She said it took hold of her, would not let go, and she had to keep working with children with cancer no matter how hard it was. "There are days when I don't want to come to work. I can't face it anymore. It's too draining. Then I get here, and I realize I could never stop doing what I do. I'm called to do it: it's in my blood and I could never do anything else." She told him that she and all her nurses were in therapy.

He could not imagine the courage it took to walk into those rooms smiling, happy, and cheerful doing everything within your power to make one more day fun and pleasant for a child you knew might die. He was affected by the pathos of pediatric oncology, but he was lifted up by the knowledge there were people in the world like the Pedi oncology nurses who demonstrated to him what caring, and empathy could do in the face of the worst of circumstances.

During his summer jobs in medical school, Dave learned that the real job of health care is done by nurses. As he progressed through his internship, his respect and admiration for nurses continued to grow. Doctors give the orders, but nurses carry out those orders, and many times good nurses question bad orders or see that good orders are instituted. He learned there is no substitute for a good nurse, and patient outcomes often depended on the quality of nursing care. The work of the Pedi oncology nurses further bolstered his opinion that nursing is a calling that requires dedication and a depth of empathy beyond many physicians.

Midway through his Pedi rotation something happened that caused everything inside him to collapse. It was as if he were hollowed out and filled with a vacuum nothing rushed in to replace. He was a little sick from the clinic because he had been seeing a lot of children with cold and flu symptoms, so maybe that had something to do with it, but it hit all the doctors and nurses on the ward just as hard.

She was simply a beautiful little girl with bouncing curls, an infectious smile, a joyful laugh, an inquisitive mind, and an engaging personality. She was observant and bright, so she had to know everything; constantly asking, "what dat? what dat noise? what dat for?" She refused to stay in her bed, dragging her parents all over the ward, clutching her beloved teddy bear in her left arm. The nurses fell in love with her immediately and indulged her every whim. They let her stay in the nurses' station sitting in their laps while they did their charting, and followed them on their rounds, always clutching her teddy bear in her left arm. She talked to everyone, brightening their day with her special glow.

She also had a lump in her left lower leg that was malignant, and she had been referred to University Hospital's Pediatric Oncology Service by her pediatrician for amputation of the leg and a work-up for metastasis. It would turn out to be an osteosarcoma, a type of cancer that occurs in the bones of children. There was a good survival rate if it had not metastasized, but only a one in three chance of survival if it had. She had been admitted for a pre-op evaluation before her surgery. She went through the work-up without complaint, never letting go of her teddy bear the whole time.

She did not just charm the nurses, she charmed everyone on the floor, including Dave. He never knew her name because everyone, including her parents, called her Little One, Sweetheart, or some other term of endearment. She must have been about five. She did not know she had cancer or that the doctors were going to cut her leg off, she just thought the whole thing was a great adventure. Her parents knew, but they maintained a brave face, smiled, and played with her as if nothing was wrong.

When she left for surgery the next morning, everyone was there to see her off. She was clutching her teddy bear and smiling although he could tell she was a little confused by all the attention. It was when she came back from recovery that she tore Dave's heart into pieces. She was sedated but still holding her teddy bear as she was wheeled down the hall on a gurney. When he looked at her tiny form lying on the gurney, he saw the outline of one leg under the sheet but on the other side: nothing. He knew that if the work-up showed the cancer had metastasized, she only had a one in three chance of living, and even if she had no mets, she faced a long rehab with PT, pain, and an ever-changing prosthesis as she grew. She would never be able to run and play as she had on the ward before the surgery, instead she would face a lifetime of wearing and managing a prosthesis. That was a lot to ask of a child: if she survived: of course, dying was a lot more to ask of a child.

Veteran oncology nurses who had seen it all and been hardened by years of exposure to children with cancer were crying, as were the poor child's parents as they followed the gurney. Seeing her tiny body on the gurney still clutching her teddy bear with only one leg, hit him like a hard punch to the gut.

As he drove home that day, the same questions kept repeating in his head. *How do you tell a child when she wakes up with no leg that the doctors had to cut her leg off? How do you tell a child she has cancer, and cancer is why they had to cut her leg off when she has no idea what cancer is? How does a child process that? How do you explain the pain she has now, and the ghost pain she will have later? She thought she was on a wonderful adventure, but now her leg was gone, and she is in horrific pain. How do you explain that to her? How do you tell her she may die? How do you explain death to a child?*

A sickening sadness engulfed him in an aura of gloom. When he got to his apartment, he lay on his bed gazing up at the ceiling. *What malevolent force does something like that to such a wonderful child? What underlying evil caused his sister and this exceptional child to suffer and for what purpose? Does being a doctor even make a difference when you aren't able to do anything about things like this?* Dave was emotionally drained and psychologically exhausted. It had been a long, hard ten months, he was at the end of himself, and the little girl's case had pushed him near the edge.

It felt as if he were sinking into the mattress with an unseen weight pressing down on him. That is the way Sharon found him when she got to his apartment after her trip. She knew something was wrong because he was lying on his bed fully dressed and he did not acknowledge her, but just kept staring at the ceiling as she sat on the bed next to him. "Are you alright?"

"It was a rough day." He sat up and put his arms around his knees. "Something happened today that broke my heart. I can't tell you about it, I can't talk about it, I can't even think about it, but I will never be able to forget it. I have about a half dozen things like that inside me now. Things I can't talk about or think about, but things I can never forget. Things that hurt my heart and left a permanent mark on my psyche. I don't know how many more things like that I can take. You just get numb. Maybe that's what has to happen: you get numb so you don't feel the pain anymore and you can deal with anything without it hurting."

"I don't want you numb, I don't want your heart hurt, or your psyche marked. I want this internship over." She knew he was on a raw emotional ledge, and she was afraid he was going to fall off the cliff. "Dave, you are burned out."

"It's warm out even though it is late, and I haven't been in the water for months. Let's go to the pool. Put your bikini on, and let's go wash these blues away." There was more sadness in his eyes than she had ever seen, and a feeling of despair surrounded him like a dark cloud hovering over him.

She knew it was bad, really bad, but she knew just what he needed. The feel of her body against him lifted some of the black fog shrouding his soul, but something intangible kept pulling him down and he could not shake it off. It was a darkness that covered his being. He needed to escape it, but he did not know how. "Can you wear the white bikini?

I know you said it was old, and you would never wear it again, but I realize I loved you in that bikini."

Sharon leaned back from him. "I think there is more lust than love associated with that white bikini, but OK, if that will cheer you up." He grabbed a couple of beers, water, towels, and they headed for the pool.

He threw the stuff he was carrying on a table, kicked off his flops, dove in, and began to swim laps. She stood by watching him for a while, then pulled two lounge chairs together, took her cover-up off, and laid down. She had seen this kind of behavior from him before when he was really stressed, but she had never seen him sad like this. Even when he was stressed, he was usually happy, upbeat, and positive. She opened herself a beer and waited for him to finish his baptismal and purification ritual. It was a glorious spring evening with a clear power blue sky heralding the onset of night. The flowers in the landscaping around the apartments were in bloom and the warm air was fragrant. She watched him swimming in the sparkling transparent water for a while, then looked around to see a few people she recognized from last summer.

Finally, he got out of the pool, walked over to her, picked up his towel, and dried off. "I needed that swim desperately. What I really need is to be sailing on a day like this, but I don't have a boat or an ocean, or to be spring skiing, but I don't have a mountain."

She stood up in front of him and put her arms around his neck. "Poor little boy. You don't have a boat to sail; you don't have a mountain to ski; you don't have any toys to play with."

Seeing her in the white bikini reminded him of the day he realized he loved her, that now seemed so long ago it was like another lifetime. They lay on their lounge chairs sipping their beers and watched the fading of the perfect spring evening. He looked at the glistening clear water of the pool, the half-dozen attractive people sitting around it, the cloudless sky, and all the vividly colored blossoms. He looked at her lying next to him with one knee cocked up and one arm over her head in the skimpy white bikini that barely covered her drinking a beer.

It occurred to him it was a Thursday, a "Sweet Thursday" like Steinbeck described in his book.

This can't be the same world I was in a few hours ago. I'm lying beside a pool with a beautiful woman, while a special little girl is lying in a hospital bed with only one leg in horrific pain. How can those two things exist in the same space and time? Did all that really happen this morning or was it just a bad dream, a nightmare? Is this Sweet Thursday real or is it just a fantasy, a fabrication of reality?

He thought about the veteran oncology nurses crying over the little girl and he realized they were reacting appropriately. They knew how to deal with tragedy: they dealt with it all the time. They were getting in touch with their emotions and appropriately expressing them. It was a terribly sad thing, so they cried. By getting in touch with their emotions and expressing them, they were able to cope with it in a healthy, healing way. He choked up, but he didn't cry. He was not able to get in touch with his emotions because that was too painful. He stuffed his feelings and buried them with denial along with all the other things he had dealt with during his internship. They were buried deep inside him in a toxic waste dump that was corroding his psyche from within. It required all his psychological energy to keep the toxicity at bay, but the little girl's plight had overloaded the system, broken the seal on the gate, and allowed it all to flood out.

Her case made him realize he could not continue to deal with tragedy by denying it. He had to talk to someone, deal with his feelings, and heal. He had to have the courage to accept the pain, regardless of how much it hurt. Terrible things happened to good people. He knew that intellectually, but not emotionally. That is why he had become a doctor, to help good people when terrible things happened to them. That is what oncology nurses do, they help good people when terrible things happen to them. Understanding that emotionally was like lifting the dark cloud from his soul. He had forgotten his primary directive: try to help but do no harm.

Both worlds were real; they were one world, his world, the world he had chosen. The world he had to become comfortable in if he was going to be a doctor. His naiveté and idealism had prevented him from seeing things clearly in a mature and realistic way. It had taken a little girl losing her leg and some oncology nurses to teach him how to cope: not by stuffing and denying his emotions to avoid the pain, but by having the courage to face the pain, embrace his emotions, and express them in a healthy, healing way.

Sharon had finished her beer and was lying back with her eyes closed, enjoying the fragrant air and soft caress of the sinking spring sun as their part of that world rotated away from it. Dave interrupted her lack of thought. "I want to talk. I understand a lot now that I didn't until today. Really until just now. I was afraid this year was going to change me, and it has. But today I realized I was changing myself by how I was dealing with the things I encountered at the hospital. I dealt with something today I couldn't stuff or deny, it was just too sad. It made me realize I need to talk to someone to get help with expressing my feelings, healing my wounds, and dealing with the pain. I think every training program should make therapy available to their house officers; in fact, I think house officers should be required to meet with a therapist on a regular basis to keep them from being permanently damaged by the stress and emotional duress they deal with on a daily basis. I have no doubt I have some form of post-traumatic stress syndrome. I think everyone who goes through this kind of training ends up with a kind of PTSD. If I can't find a therapist to see me, I will find one who wants to do a paper on stressed out interns."

"I agree. Remember, I asked you if you had someone you could talk to when we first met." She sat up and looked at him lying beside her.

"I have difficulty dealing with death, trying to understand it, and feeling helpless because I can't do anything about it. I also struggle with trying to understand why terrible things happen. I must learn to accept that terrible things happen, forget about why they happen, and try to help. That's my job as a doctor, to try to help; try to help and do no harm. That also means not harming myself to the point where I can't help anyone, including myself. Do all you can to help, then acknowledge and move on to the next one, because there is no end to the suffering."

Sharon felt a sense of relief. "I am so glad you're back to being yourself again."

"Don't think I am the same person I was because I am not. Before this internship, I was a doctor in name only. I had the degree, but I wasn't a doctor: now I am. It was one hell of a rough road to get here, but it is absolutely necessary for anyone who wants to be a doctor to travel that road. I lost my way on the road for a while but today I found it again. The road came close to consuming me until I remembered why I was on the road in the first place." Dave stood up and held out his hand to her. "Come on, I want to get back in the water."

They swam for a while, then Dave got out, and stood in front of the ladder to watch Sharon get out. She stopped and stood on the ladder looking at him. "What is it with you and water; in the shower, in the bathtub, in the pool; they all have the same erotic effect on you."

He got a towel and handed her one. "Water is my natural habitat, and I thrive in it or on it, liquid or frozen. Let's dry off and go in. We can listen to some music, order a pizza for dinner, and then let nature take its course."

Her bikini was off as soon as he had her in the door of his apartment. They were driven by a hunger to leave an emotional day behind them, and they devoured each other as the long shadows of early evening spread through the room.

It was dark, they were lying on the floor, the music had stopped, and they were letting the night wash over them through the window. Neither of them said anything. There was nothing to say, nothing needed to be said; they had said it all with their lovemaking, and they had woven a spell they did not want to break. From the very first time they had sex on the night they met, their lovemaking had been over-powering and all consuming. Now, almost a year later, it had only grown more intensity.

At last, Sharon sat up. "We need to shower and order the pizza. You have to work tomorrow, and I am leaving for Caroline's wedding. I wish you were going with me. Not having a plus-one is an invitation for a lot of unwanted attention. I have been to enough weddings to know how it goes. There will be a lot of single guys there looking to hook up with someone."

Caroline was getting married in her hometown and Jake was driving Audrey, who was Caroline's maid of honor, Helen and Sharon, who were both bridesmaids, to the wedding for the rehearsal and rehearsal dinner on Friday. The wedding and reception were on Saturday, and they would drive back on Sunday morning so Sharon would be back in time to meet Dave. Sunday was match day.

His last few days on the Pedi wards were uneventful and on Sunday morning he went to the administrative offices to check the main bulletin board for the match list. Harvin matched with UCLA and George matched with the Tulane program at Charity Hospital in New Orleans. He called Harvin. "Let's have a match party tonight at the park house. Nothing big, just get together and celebrate." When he got to his apartment, letters from USC and UCLA were waiting for him. He was accepted by both programs, so he was on his way to UCLA for his Internal Medicine residency.

When she opened the door, he grabbed her. "Westwood, Baby, Hollywood straight away." He spun around with her until they fell into a beanbag together, but she could not stay there and got up to swirl around the room again.

"I can't believe it's really happening. We're going to California." She stopped. "Oh my God, I need tell my mother. I have to call her. Calling her and telling her I'm moving to California is going to be tough. If you have any doubts about how I feel about you, understand that I'm going against my own mother to be with you." She turned in a circle with her arms out. "I don't want to call her now and spoil how I feel. I'll call her later."

"Don't worry. I'll charm her." Dave got up and tried to hold her again, but she spun away from him. "You don't know my mother."

"How was the wedding?" He gave up and sat down in a bean bag.

Her mood changed. "Fine, we had a nice drive up with Jake. Audrey's wedding is next, but I am not going alone. I will ride up with Helen for the rehearsal and rehearsal dinner, you can drive up the next morning after you get off, sleep in my room until the wedding, then we can drive back after the reception. That's another reason you should have no doubts about me. The groomsman I was paired with was handsome, charming, and witty." She joined him in the bean bag. "He had it all; looks, intelligence, personality. He graduated from Princeton with Ron. My mother would have thought he was the perfect man for me." She paused. "He invited me to his room after the reception."

"Really! I hate jerks like that. He knew you were with someone, and he still went after you?" Dave sat up in the bean bag and looked at her.

She looked down. "I told him I was seeing someone, and it was serious, but he came on strong from the beginning, telling me how beautiful I was, and keeping my Champagne glass full. He said we could enjoy a good time together and you would never know. He was a real player like a lot of the guys I dated before Bar and before you."

"How do I know you didn't sleep with him?" Dave could not control his jealousy.

She looked at him intently. "If I did, why would I tell you about him? We're together. I will tell you if that ever changes." She stood up. She loved him. She could not bring herself to say it yet because it scared the hell out of her to admit it, even to myself, but she loved him. She had to find out before she changed her entire life by moving to California with him if he did his residency there, but she knew now. She knew she wanted to spend her life with him. "I have to go home and get ready for the party. I will see you in an hour. Try to get your head screwed on straight by then."

She answered the door and broke out laughing. "Great idea. It'll only take me a minute to change. Helen and Linda are in the kitchen." She ran back upstairs. He was dressed in the same T-shirt and jeans he wore the night they met. He found Helen and a dark-haired woman in her early thirties sitting at the table in the kitchen. Even though her attire was feminine, her hair was short, and so were her unpolished nails.

"Dave, this is Linda." The woman nodded to him as he sat down with them. "Linda moved into Caroline's room while we were at the wedding. She is a flight attendant I have been working with since Sharon started bidding around your call schedule. We are going to get an apartment together when you and Sharon move to California."

Sharon joined them in the kitchen and Helen laughed when she saw her. "They're wearing the same things they wore the night they met, like they were in high school. This party is to celebrate the guys matching with their internship programs. Dave was accepted for a residency at UCLA and they're moving to LA together."

Linda looked admiringly at Sharon. "I can see why he was all over you."

Helen stood up. "She was all over him too, I mean literally all over him. Are you two ready to go, now."

"The way she looks, I'm surprised they're even going to the party." Linda continued to admire Sharon.

Sharon held her hand out to Dave. "Let's go. I want a glass of wine, I want to dance, and I want to celebrate." She looked back at Linda. "Then I want to do what we did the night we met." She pulled him up and started for the door.

"I'm on it. I got it. Wine, dance, celebrate, and" Dave gave Helen and Linda a Cheshire Cat grin, "fornicate. Come on ladies, let's go."

They walked to the house next door with Helen and Linda following behind. "Look at them. They are so cute, it's disgusting. I am going to miss her terribly. I'm going to miss all three of them, but I am going to miss her the most. I want to dislike Dave for taking her away from me but look how happy she is. When she came back from finding out he was accepted by UCLA, she danced up the stairs singing California Dreaming. There used to be a sadness about her, and she was never completely happy, but since she met him, it is like the dark cloud that surrounded her lifted, and her inner light began to shine through."

Linda nodded at them. "I guess that's true love."

Helen looked at them and mused. "I wonder what it is like to feel like that about someone?"

"I don't know, but I would like to find out." Linda replied, they looked at each other, walked on, and caught up with Sharon and Dave on the porch of the other house. Dave turned to them. "Stop lagging, it's party time. We need to get on with the wine, dance, and celebration parts."

"I know, so you can get to the last part." Helen laughed as Dave opened the door.

"I'm surprised you didn't skip all the other parts and go straight to the last part to begin with. I know I would have." The last thing Linda said was lost on Sharon and Dave, but not on Helen. She looked at Linda again, more intently this time.

As they walked through the door they heard, "I'm gonna miss your ass, brother. You taking that little girl with you?" Henry had started to celebrate early.

"I'm leaving your ass behind brother, and this little girl is gonna make that California trip with me." Dave looked over his shoulder at Sharon. "You think I would leave that behind?"

"I am not a 'that'. I think if someone wants to make it to the last part of tonight, like we talked about, they better not call me a 'that'." Sharon frowned at Dave.

Harvin and Connie sauntered up to the group and Harvin did a little buggy. "Won't you get hip to this timely tip, when you take that California trip, Get your kicks on Route Sixty-Six".

George joined them. He was more animated and excited than Dave had ever seen him. "Not everyone is going to California. Some of us aren't getting above our raising and are staying right here in the sunny Southland."

Sigrid pulled on Henry's arm. "What did he say about raisins?"

"Not raisins, Sigrid, raising."

"What is his raising? What does it mean?"

"He is speaking Appalachian. There is no English translation."

Dave, Harvin, and Henry went to the dining room for drinks, and George went back to the front room with the women. Henry told them that Sigrid was finally moving in with him. His family had funded an extension on her grant, and he promised her she could fly home anytime she wanted. Harvin suggested they take their vacations together next year in January and meet somewhere to ski. Henry volunteered his family's lodge in Colorado where he and Dave skied when they were in college. They got beers and wine for the girls then headed for the front room.

Mike and Janice arrived amid the chaos. Mike sat down next to Sharon, smirked, and said. "Dave's not doing his residency here, so you're not moving in together, and that means you're not exclusive anymore. When is he leaving for LA? I don't want your bed to get cold." What he said caught Sharon completely off guard, then she remembered what she told him the night he showed up at her house drunk, and she was flabbergasted.

"Unless of course you want to hookup before he leaves. He going to be gone anyway, so why waste time." He smiled, leaned back, and put his arm around her.

"Really Mike, the woman you're dating is right there," she pushed his arm off of her, and pointed to Janice who was sitting on another couch chattering away, "and the man I'm dating, who is supposed to be your friend, is in the next room, and you're not just hitting on me, you're making a move on me."

He smiled, "Like I said, why waste time. You said I would be the first guy you hooked up with after Dave. Well, Dave is basically gone, and a woman like you doesn't sleep alone for long. It's time for you to move on from Dave to the next guy; me."

Her mind was reeling, she did not know what to say, then it hit her. Mike did something to keep Dave from doing his residency here? He screwed his friend because he wanted to screw her? He interfered with Dave's life and as a result interfered with her life, because you want to sleep with her? Like a lot of men, he was a devious bastard, and he manipulated her life in order to have sex with her? "I going to LA, Mike. I'm transferring to LAX. I'm never going to be with you, and I never intended to hook up with you. I just wanted to get your drunk ass out of my house that night, so I could go to sleep. Like I told you then, and like I'm telling you now, I'm with Dave."

The smug look on Mike's face disappeared, and it turned bright red. "I didn't tell Dave about that night, and I'm not going to tell him about this either, because I don't want to be responsible for what he would to you. But stay away from me, Mike, or I will tell him." She nodded toward the opening to the room. Dave walked in, handed Sharon her wine, and put his hand out for her. She stood up, took Dave's hand, scowled at Mike, and the three couples walked away.

Dave had not spoken to Mike or acknowledged him in any way since another intern on the medicine service told him what Mike was doing. Mike was telling the house staff he worked with that Dave was a sexual predator who could not be trusted with women. He was saying Dave was not fit to be a doctor because he would use his position as a physician to exploit women. The intern told Dave it appeared that Mike was doing everything possible to make sure Dave did not stay at University Hospital for his residency. After Dave found out what Mike was doing, he considered confronting Mike about it, but it was too late, the damage was done: Dave was not staying at University Hospital for his residency. Mike could have influenced his recommendations and damaged his chances of getting in one of the California programs, but that had not happened, so he let it go.

He had a problem with his Medicine grade in medical school, and that was why he could not apply for a straight medicine internship. He wondered at the time if Mike was involved in what happened in some way. Now he was sure he was, but Mike had actually facilitated two events in Dave's life in a positive way. He would not have met Sharon if he had done a straight medicine internship, because he would not have matched with the program here, and he would not be on his way to California with her, if Mike had not sabotaged his chances of staying here.

They went to the back room and Harvin explained his idea of meeting to ski every January and Henry added they could use his family's ski lodge in Colorado. Sharon wanted to know if there was enough room to include Audrey, Jake, Caroline, and Ron. Henry responded, "There's six bedrooms, so there's plenty of room."

"Six bedrooms!" Sigrid looked shocked. "That is not a ski lodge, that's a chateau. How many other places like that does your family own?"

Henry tried to hedge, "My parents and my aunt and uncle own homes."

But Sigrid pressed him. "How many others?"

Henry mumbled, "Granny owns a ranch in Texas, a beach house in the Keys, the ski lodge in Colorado, and a place in Dallas."

Sigrid was not going to be deterred. "How big is the ranch?"

"A little over twenty thousand acres." Henry said quietly.

"Twenty thousand acres! The beach house and the ranch house, they are as big as the ski lodge, and what about your grandmother's house?" Sigrid was incredulous.

"No, actually they're bigger." Henry answered sheepishly. "The ranch house is a copy of an antebellum plantation house, the beach house is really a complex in a large compound, and my grandmother's house is a mansion on Turtle Creek in Dallas."

Sigrid looked hard at Henry. She was overwhelmed. "It does not matter to you that so many are homeless, yet your family has so many big houses and so much land? I knew you were rich Henry, but I did not know your family was that rich."

"Does it make a difference?" Henry asked with a worried look.

She paused, "I am not sure."

Henry tried to put his arm around her, but she pulled away. "You might as well know it all. There is an apartment in Paris my sister lives in and one in New York City my cousin lives in. My other cousin lives in San Francisco in a house on Knob Hill. There is a yacht with a captain, cook, and crew berthed in the compound in Florida. Sigrid, my family once owned a great deal of land, and that land has oil on it. The family sold most of the land but kept the mineral rights, so there is a considerable annual income from those oil leases, and we all have trust funds created from the money generated by selling the land. I told you all this when we met"

Sigrid moved away from him. "I am not sure I know who you really are, Henry. You are a member of the wealthy, landed class I despise, but you keep that side of yourself hidden from me."

Harvin changed the subject. "Okay, we're committed. We meet at Henry's to ski in January."

"You bet," Dave answered, and they nodded in agreement.

The interchange between Sigrid and Henry had changed the mood considerably. Connie stood up. "Some of us have to work tomorrow, so let's go Harvin."

"Next year we will all ski together in Colorado, right." Harvin said as they left.

Henry stood up with Sigrid. "I guess it's time to take my shield maiden home. We'll see you guys when you get back from California."

"I am not a shield maiden. You are an earl with all your houses and money. An earl would not have a mere shield maiden for a lover. He would have a Viking princess, but you had better be a good earl and you had better help others with all your money, or you will not have a princess or even a shield maiden." She said goodbye to Sharon and Dave, and they left.

Dave tried to get up, but Sharon pulled him back down. He looked at her and her top was unbuttoned. "There are still people here. Someone might walk in on us."

She stood up, walked to the door, and closed it. "I don't care." She walked back, pushed him down on his back, straddled him and began to undo his belt.

"Did you plan this?" He helped her get his pants off.

She slipped out of her thong and sat down on him with her skirt up around her waist. "Not until I saw you in that stupid T-shirt, your tight rear in those jeans, and I remembered how hot I was for you that night." She leaned down and put her breast in front of his face and he buried himself in her softness. "Dave, I'm very happy, and I want to do what we did that night right here where it started."

He locked his arms around her, rolled over on top of her and did just that until she cried out, grabbed the cushions with both hands, dug her fingers into them, then beat them with her fist. He drove her into the cushions before the sound had time to die away, as she grabbed them again to hold on.

Walking back to her house Dave mused. "Poor Henry, he has always been so careful about who he dated. Now he is in love with someone who has a problem with him being wealthy."

"She loves him despite his wealth, not because of it, and that has him totally off balance. I understand Henry. He was afraid he would be loved for his wealth, not for who he is. I was afraid I would be loved for my looks, and not for who I am." Sharon took his hand.

"But Sigrid sees Henry's wealth as a deterrent." Dave countered.

"The kind of wealth Henry has will open doors for her she never dreamed existed. She is still trying to get her head around it. She doesn't understand how that kind of money can help her do whatever she wants to do, and more than she ever conceived of doing."

They walked on to the house, went upstairs, and straight in bed. Dave still had a day to rest and relax before he started his rotation in the Nursery.

Chapter 12

The Bell Tolls for Sharon

M ajor problems in the Nursery were managed by the residents. Fetal alcohol syndrome was terrible, and drug addicted babies went through withdrawal, had seizures, and often suffered permanent brain damage. Dave managed a few cases of babies with Down syndrome and other mild birth defects, but mainly he admitted normal healthy infants who needed little care.

He did however, admit premature infants that were so small and fragile he was afraid to touch them, but his supervising resident helped him calculate the micro doses of meds, oxygen, and fluids necessary to maintain the tiny babies. Some did not make it, succumbing to hyaline membrane disease or other problems, but many of those preemies barely had the organ base necessary for survival, so each one he saved seemed like a miracle and overshadowed the ones he lost.

Dave's shifts in the Nursery were busy. He made rounds with the students and his resident in the morning, admitted newborn babies, answered calls from the Nursery to handle problems, and was present to take the baby at C-sections.

When he encountered something troubling, he applied cognitive thinking, replacing what he was thinking with positive thoughts about skiing or sailing. When he was off, he applied cognitive behavior, swimming laps until he purged the stress-related toxin from his body. He found a psychiatry resident to have lunch with on a regular basis who listened to him as he talked out his most troubling issues.

Everything was going smoothly as they prepared for their trip to LA. Sharon accepted the place UCLA's Graduate School of Business offered her, and notified them she was going to continue flying. She was transferring to LAX in July. With their salaries, their savings, and the financial aid she qualified for because of her academic record, they had enough money for the move, her grad school expenses, and a yearly ski vacation with their friends. She could continue flying to take advantage of the income, excellent benefits, travel privileges, and still pursue an MBA in Marketing. By attending classes year-round, she could back fill what she missed by working, and by flying only sixteen to eighteen hours a week, she could bid around her classes. She was in control of her life now and she intended to exert that control. She drew up a blueprint for her future, a vision board, and she was going to follow that vision to build the future she had designed for herself.

The week before they left for LA, Dave was at the hospital, and she was getting ready for a trip when her phone rang. She did not recognize the number but answered anyway. He immediately launched into his usual manipulative tactics and gaslighting. A cold hard knot formed in her chest. His smooth cultured, boarding school voice triggered the memory of him smashing his fist into her face: the pain, the humiliation, and the degradation. She remembered hitting the floor after he knocked her down, slumping over, covering her face with her arms, and cowering as he stood over her with his fist cocked to hit her again. But instead, he grabbed one of her arms, pulled it away, and slapped her around her head and face as he berated her for thinking she could break up with him. The horror of that moment resurfaced in vivid images in her brain as he droned on, telling her how sorry he was, but it was not his fault. It had been transference because of the stress he was under in medical school. It was her fault he hit her because she did not understand, and she provoked him by telling him she was leaving him. She made him lash out because of the pain she caused him by threatening to break up with him. But none of it mattered now. That was all behind them, and he was coming back to do his residency at University Hospital. Her heart stopped, a trembling fear gripped her, she could not breathe, and the mindless rush of panic seized her.

He droned on telling her he was coming back, and they could be together again. He repeated it mechanically several times. "We are two superior people who are meant for each other. Our destiny is to be together. Ordinary people are beneath us. We are exceptional and exceptional people belong with other exceptional people." Then he completely went off the rails, "You belong to me. It is your destiny to be with me. Do you really think you can escape that destiny? You can't, because it is my destiny to be with you. You're mine!"

He was totally unhinged! She could not speak even if he had given her a chance, but he went on without a pause. He promised her how wonderful things were going to be. He would lavish dinners, flowers, and gifts on her. He would make sure she had everything she desired.

The cold hard knot in her chest sank like a stone to the pit of her stomach. The black specter of Bartholomew Augustus Reynolds suddenly cast its long dark shadow in the bright sunlight of her new life. She had been sure it was over when she made it clear to him in no uncertain terms she was not transferring to Boston, and moving there when he came for her on his vacation. She made it crystal clear to him she never wanted to see him again and hung up on him.

His sophisticated voice with perfect grammar, enunciation, and pronunciation impressed her when they first met, but now it terrified her. She had let a sociopath into her life, and now he's out of his mind! It was that voice that frightened her, that deep melodious hypnotic voice, and the way he used it to manipulate her, to coerce her, and she feared the intelligence behind the voice; the intelligence behind his cold calculating emotionless personality. She also feared the power behind his intelligence and personality: his father. But she could not think about that now. She had to get to the airport and not be late for her flight. The cold hard frozen stone that sat in the pit of her stomach radiated a chill throughout her body producing a frost that permeated her whole being. She hung up on him without saying a word and ran to her car as if she was trying to run away from him: to run away from his intelligence, his calculating manipulative personality, and that voice. She had to get away from his voice.

The frost produced a quivering in her core, but the quivering began to subside, and the cold stone in the pit of her stomach began to dissipate as she drove. Without his voice in her head, she settled down, and came to grips with reality. That voice had caused an irrational mindless fear to grip her, but now that she was over the shock of hearing it, she regained control. What was she afraid of? He was in Boston. When he comes back for his residency, she will be in California. What is she going to do, follow her to California? His father has no influence there. It's a different state, thousands of miles away, controlled by a different political party. All she needs to do is leave for LA before he returns, and if he comes back before she leaves, she simply needs to avoid him.

Her fear slowly melted with the heat of anger and then burst into the flames of rage. How dare he interpose his vile toxic darkness into the light of her happy new life. For a brief fleeting moment, she considered telling Dave he called her and was coming back, but she was ashamed of even having such a thought. She knew what Dave would do and the prospect of that was frightening. No, he will show up here and she will be on her way to California. He will be left with his nose pressed up against the glass watching her taillights disappear into the West, and she will be out of his reach forever.

When she returned from her trip, dozens of red roses were waiting for her with a big box of chocolates and a giant stuffed teddy bear. She recalled the "love bombing" that went on when they first met: the flowers, the dinners, and the flattering compliments in his charmingly captivating voice. It had all seemed so wonderful at the time. He is the one-eyed jack in a deck of cards that only shows one side of its face and keeps the other side hidden. But she had seen the twisted and grotesque other side of his face. Did he think she could forget that face? The face she saw when he was standing over her screaming at her and slapping her repeatedly.

The phone rang and she knew it was him. He was calling her as soon as she returned from her trip. He had her schedule. She did not know how he managed to get it, but he had it. Knowing that caused the chill to return briefly, but it was quickly vanquished and replaced by anger again. She seriously considered answering and telling him if he tried to see her, the man she was with now would beat him to a bloody pulp. She did not need to do that. Her future was planned, and that future did not include Bartholomew Augustus Reynolds in any way, shape, or form. She was through with him. She let the phone ring while she threw the flowers, chocolates, and bear in the garbage. She deleted the message without listening to it. A few days later they left for LA.

Sharon knew the flight crew and there were seats in first-class, so the first-class flight attendant moved them up, brought them two glasses of Champagne, and continued to refill their glasses throughout the flight. They arrived at LAX, retrieved their bags, picked up the rental car, and drove to the UCLA campus. It was a Sunday but there were still a few people in the Administration Building. They met with a young man who reviewed Sharon's file and had her complete the forms she needed to start classes in September. She asked him about a place to live and he told her most students lived on campus because housing in the area was so expensive.

At the hospital they went to the administration offices to pick up the forms Dave needed. Then they went to a medicine floor where they found some of the house medicine staff in the doctor's station. They acted annoyed when Dave introduced himself until the twenty something young men in the station saw Sharon; they became very attentive, introducing themselves to her, ignoring Dave, and offering her a place to sit, and something to drink. Sharon noticed the women in the station continued to ignore them. Dave asked where they should look for a place to live and a resident told him further out the Santa Monica freeway, near the San Diego freeway because it would take him to Torrance for his rotations there. The resident was nice looking, polite, well mannered, as he talked to Sharon, not Dave. "There is a sweet spot where most of us live between the expensive stuff in Westwood and the equally expensive places at the beach. You need to get a rental agent, or you'll waste a lot of time trying to look for something on your own."

He asked if they were married. Sharon answered, "No," without further elaboration, so he pressed the point by reversing the question. "Do you already live here?"

Sharon left him hanging by saying, "I'm going to grad school here." He smiled at her and ushered them out walking beside her with Dave trailing behind.

By the time they located the hotel, he was dead tired, but she was energized by being in such a glamorous place. They were surrounded by famous neighborhoods; Bel Air, Brentwood, Beverly Hills, and Holly-wood; with streets named Sunset Boulevard, Santa Monica Boulevard, Wilshire Boulevard, Hollywood, Vine, and Mulholland Drive. They had both grown up in small Southern towns and although they had lived in large cities in the South, big cities in the South were not LA with street names connected with fame and celebrity.

Their hotel in Santa Monica was within walking distance of the beach and pier. When they got to the room Dave took his clothes off and climbed onto the bed. "I have to take a little nap." Sharon reminded him that they needed to eat. "We will eat when I wake up. I'm only going to take a short nap." He slept straight through until the next morning.

He woke up early. "God, I am starving."

"You forgot to eat last night." She was already up.

"I haven't felt this rested and relaxed for a long time. How long did I sleep?" He got out of bed and reached for her.

"Stop that, we have to find a place to live." Sharon was trying to dress, and everything she put on, he tried to take off. "Being rested and relaxed makes you too frisky. Get dressed so we can have breakfast and call a rental agent." She put her arms around his neck and kissed him lightly. "We have work to do."

They walked to a diner near the hotel and after breakfast, he began calling rental agents. On the fourth call, he found someone. The agent told them to enjoy their morning and she would pick them up at their hotel at one o'clock.

"Rodeo Drive," was all she said, and she was out the door.

They drove to one of the most famous shopping streets in the world and walked along widow shopping until Sharon found a stylish dress shop and pulled him in. They were dressed in jeans, T-shirts, and sandals, unlike the other shoppers who were in expensive couture. She found a dress she liked, and a straight-faced unsmiling clerk led Sharon to a dressing room saying, "You seem rather rural. You're not from LA, are you?"

Sharon came out of the dressing room and showed Dave the dress. "Where are you going to wear a dress like that?"

"I have something in mind." She looked at him knowingly, then turned to the clerk. "I'll take it. It is going to need a few alterations; can you have it ready in a week?"

"Of course." The clerk finally smiled.

They left the shop and Sharon took Dave's arm. "Now it's your turn. How old are your suits? Let me guess, you bought them when you were in college, so they are at least five or six years old. You need a new suit, and this is the place to get it."

They found an exclusive men's shop, and she led him in smiling at the older gentleman who welcomed them. "He is looking for a suit." The man explained they did custom-tailored suits, but they did have a few off-the-rack suits from top designers in the back. He took them to a rack of fine suits on the back wall and pulled a few in Dave's coat size. "The problem will be the pants. His shoulders and chest are broad, but his waist is much smaller, so the pants that come with the coat won't fit him."

"I like him that way. Can you alter the pants to fit?" She flashed him one of her alluring smiles.

"I am a tailor, and I can tell you if I alter the pants that come with the jacket to fit him, they won't look right. I could swap the pants with a suit with a smaller coat size."

"Oh, could you? That would be great. I like the dark blue one with the fine pinstripe. It brings out the blue in his eyes."

"You have excellent taste. That is an exceptionally fine suit. I will do it for such a lovely young woman. Is he your husband?" The man took the coat from one suit and the pants from another identical suit in a smaller coat size and ushered Dave to a dressing room.

"No. He's, my lover." She smiled mischievously.

"Normally I would not do this, but I cannot deny such a beautiful woman. I am an Italian, and we Italians understand love. You can wait here while I mark the suit." He opened a dressing room door for Dave and sat her down in a chair nearby.

"Ciao, Bella," the man said, smiling at Sharon as they left.

When they were outside the shop, Dave took her hand again. "He liked you. That suit was marked much higher than what he charged me. Now we can dress like movie stars. Is that what you wanted?"

"Little bit. I don't think we are going to find a place to eat lunch here the way we're dressed." He drove back to Santa Monica, and they walked to the pier to get hot dogs for lunch before going back to the hotel to wait for the rental agent.

A white Mercedes convertible pulled up in front of the hotel and an attractive bottle blond in her forties dressed in a tight dress and stiletto heels got out. She clicked her way into the lobby, walked straight up to Sharon, and put her hand out. "You must be Sharon. You are a beauty aren't you, but I'm not crazy about your ensemble. A piece of advice for you my dear; dress to display your best assets and with your looks you can go a long way in this town." After shaking Sharon's hand, she turned to Dave. "And you must be David. I'm Gloria. I have three apartments to show you this afternoon, and I have three more to show you tomorrow. Don't worry, I have found apartments for a lot of graduate students and doctors training at UCLA. I am sure I can find just what you are looking for." Despite her brash, brassy approach, she had an infectious smile and warm intelligent eyes.

She led them to the convertible, opened the passenger door, pulled the seat back forward, and motioned for Dave to get in the back seat. "You sit up front with me, Sharon."

Sharon turned to Dave in the back seat. "I like her already."

Gloria looked at them, smiled, shook her head, and started the car. "You really are two babes in the woods, aren't you? Well, don't worry, Gloria will take care of you."

She put on an expensive pair of sunglasses and as she put her hands on the wheel, Dave noticed a diamond watch, gold bracelets, other rings, but no wedding ring. She was quintessential LA, but she was also a quintessential professional. "You're lucky I had a couple of days open when you called. The properties I am going to show you are in your price range, they are in safe neighborhoods, have easy access to the San Diego and Santa Monica freeways, and are reasonably near the campus. The grounds are well maintained with pools. All the units have two closets in the master; a kitchen with dishwasher, disposal, and meal area; a large front room with a patio or balcony; separate tub and shower with two sinks in the bathroom; and plenty of storage. There is a laundry with washers and dryers in the building or nearby." Gloria looked at Sharon over her sunglasses and smiled warmly. "All you two kids have to do is pick one, put down a deposit, and sign the lease."

That is exactly what they did. There was not much difference between the apartments, but the buildings, landscaping, and locations varied. Sharon picked one that was a little older with mature landscaping and a charming atmosphere. The units were one story duplex cottages that resembled old Hollywood bungalows, and each one had a small, enclosed patio. The apartment complex was not as modern or as slick as some of the others they looked at, but it had an inviting cozy atmosphere. It was exactly what she pictured in her vision of her future.

When Gloria dropped them at their hotel the next day, she took her sunglasses off and looked at Sharon with slightly sad eyes. "I have another piece of advice for you, Sharon. This is a decadent town with a lot of temptations. With your looks you are going to have guys all over you offering you everything you could imagine in your wildest dreams, but what they really want to give you is what I am sure Dave gives you quite frequently. They'll promise you whatever you desire in order to use that beautiful body of yours. You may think it's the stuff dreams are made of, but it's not. It's really about money and fame exploiting beauty for sex. Don't be seduced by Hollywood and succumb to the siren calls of Babylon." She put her sunglasses back on and drove off.

As they watched her drive away Dave remarked, "I think she is speaking from experience."

"I know she is, but I've already been exposed to the type of man she's talking about. No one is going to exploit me for sex, not the wealthy, famous men I meet on the plane, and not the men I date. No one is going to use my body for their own pleasure. Never again, I learned that lesson." She smiled seductively. "I chose who gives it to me. And tonight, after you take me out to dinner and we have a little celebration, I would like for you to give it to me, and I do mean whatever I desire." She laughed at herself.

Dave booked a room for Wednesday through Friday nights at the Disneyland Hotel and a place in Newport near the beach for Saturday night. He had already booked a room in Marina Del Rey for Sunday night, so they could get to LAX early Monday morning. Sharon had never been to Disneyland, so they would spend three days at Disneyland, drive to Newport Saturday morning for two days on the beach, and back to Marina Del Rey on Sunday night to fly home on Monday.

Sharon made the dinner reservation and told Dave he had to wear a coat and tie. She made him shower and get dressed alone, then she took a long, hot bubble bath and would not let him in the bathroom while she was getting ready. He sat on the bed and waited patiently for her.

She emerged in the quintessential little black cocktail dress with black heels and posed for him with her hands on her waist. The dress and shoes displayed her long slender legs to perfection, was tight enough to accentuate her figure, and displayed a tantalizing view of her breasts. "You look fabulous."

He moved for her, but she wagged her finger at him. "We'll get to that later. The restaurant has valet parking, but it is a lovely evening. I want to park and walk." She took his arm. "Let's go. This is our town now; let's go enjoy it."

She was vibrant and luminous as she strode along the street on his arm with her head up looking straight ahead and smiling. Beautiful women were common in the area, but she still turned heads, drew attention, and even slowed traffic. When they got to the restaurant, the maître d' greeted them. "Welcome, Dr. Cameron. I have a nice table for you and the lady." He took two menus and led them to a table, pulled out Sharon's chair, fawned over her as he placed her napkin in her lap, and gave her the menu. He stood behind her as the busser brought water and the waiter arrived to introduce himself.

"Two glasses of Champagne, then give us a little time to enjoy them before you take our order. We have something to discuss." She had picked the restaurant for a reason.

When the server brought the Champagne, she reached across the table and took both of his hands in hers. "Well, are you going to ask me to marry you?"

"What!"

"I said, are you going to ask me to marry you? Do you think I would change my whole life, and move thousands of miles away from my home with you if you weren't going to marry me?"

"What!"

"Do I have to ask you to marry me?"

"Do you mean it?"

"Do you want to marry me or not?"

"Of course, I do,"

"Then ask me."

"Yes." he blurted out.

"I'm the one who is supposed to say, yes. You are the one who is supposed to ask." She squeezed his hands.

"Will you marry me, Sharon?" He choked up as he said it.

"Yes, Dave. I'll marry you. I love you and I will marry you." She finally said it out loud. Her eyes were deep glistening pools, as she looked across the table at him. He could not stand it any longer, he had wanted to hold her since he first saw her in that dress. He stood up, walked around the table, pulled her up, and kissed her. They were surprised and embarrassed by the smattering of applause that followed. He reached back for the two Champagne flutes, they clinked glasses, and took a sip.

They were holding hands across the table, when the waiter reappeared with a bottle of Dom Perignon. "Compliments of a couple who want to wish you all the best." They finished their Champagne cocktails, asked the waiter to thank their benefactors, and started on the bottle of Dom Perignon. After they finished their meal, the waiter brought the dessert menu. "For dessert, I recommend baked Alaska flambé. It will go perfectly with the Champagne." As they waited for dessert, Dave looked across the table at her and felt something immensely powerful overcome him. It was a transcendental state of perfection, joy, balance, harmony, and contentment that no language could describe and only those who have reached it can understand. In that moment he had it all, he was at the top of the mountain, the peak of his existence, the absolute reality of all his dreams and aspirations.

On the way back to the car they strolled along on the clear Southern California spring night, smelling the salty sea air off the Pacific Ocean, as happy and content as two people could be. The blood, gore, stress, fatigue, and heartache of University Hospital were far away and forgotten. It was as if they were in some distant land where nothing like that existed.

Dave woke up with a headache and a dry mouth. *All that Champagne.* He looked over at Sharon who was still sleeping tangled in the sheet and smiled as he remembered last night.

He tried to get up but that made his head hurt worse and the morning sun was pouring in through the window, setting his eyes on fire. *Coffee, I have to have coffee. Water first, then coffee, lots of water, then lots of coffee.*

He tried again and managed to struggle up to the bathroom to drink several glasses of water. Then he called for more packets of coffee. None of this disturbed Sharon's sleep, even when the house cleaner brought the extra packets of coffee she slept on, partially covered in the tangled twisted sheet.

He drank more water, started the coffee, and went through his stuff looking for aspirin. The way he felt reminded him of the mornings after a fraternity party in college. The smell of the coffee finally caused Sharon to stir, she rolled over, leaving herself mostly uncovered and exposed. "You got me drunk on Champagne and took advantage of me. Jesus, did you ever take advantage of me. You are a bad man."

He got her a glass of water, which she drank, then handed him the glass for more. "Do you have any aspirin or Tylenol?" She walked to the bathroom for more water. "God, what a wonderful night."

He poured two cups of coffee. "No, I'm depending on coffee to bring me back to life. You planned it all, didn't you? The dress, the suit; that's your wedding dress and my wedding suit. You picked the restaurant and made the reservation because you knew famous celebrities went there. You wore that dress because you knew what would happen once I had you alone. You even talked dirty to me to encourage and tease me." When she came out of the bathroom, he handed her a cup of coffee.

She took the coffee and smiled at him over the cup. "Little bit."

"Don't call me a bad man. You are a devious, cunning woman." He put his free arm around her. "You are now the future wife of the esteemed Doctor Cameron. What changed your mind?"

She looked serious and sat down on the side of the bed with her coffee. "Getting married is for us, for our future. We need to become legitimate." Sharon put the coffee cup down on the bedside table, stood up, and walked into his arms. That was not the real reason, but she could never tell him the real reason. She went to Alexander's room that night after the reception intending to spend the night with him. She had made up her mind to sleep with him. As soon as she was in his room, he kissed her, and had his hands all over her. When he started taking her dress off and maneuvering her toward the bed, she realized he did not make her feel the way Dave made her feel. He was kissing her, but it did not feel the way it felt when Dave kissed her. His touch did not excite her the way Dave's touch did. She did not feel safe, secure, and protected in his arms the way she did in Dave's. Nothing felt the way it did with Dave. It did not feel right, and she was about to have sex with him. She knew in that moment she could never kiss another man; she never wanted another man's hands on her or his arms around her; and she could never have sex with anyone but Dave. She discovered she loved him, and how much she loved him in another man's arms. She finally accepted that she wanted to marry him with another man kissing her, holding her, fondling her, and taking her dress off to have sex with her. She pulled her dress back on, left him standing there calling her a "bitch", and ran back to her room like she was running back to Dave. When she got to her room, she fell onto the bed and cried. But she could never tell him any of that.

"I love you and I want to grow old with you. I know you are nothing like my father and you would never treat me the way my father treated my mother. I must admit all my friends getting married had something to do with it too, so I planned the perfect seduction and asked you to marry me. Do you mind terribly that I did it that way?"

"Of course not, I will never forget last night." He walked her to the bed and they both sat down on the side of the bed. "But with the expense of the move, the apartment and everything, I can't buy you a ring, there'll be no honeymoon, when are we going to have time to get married, and how are we going to pay for a wedding?"

She nuzzled his neck. "I want two simple, matching bands of gold. I'll buy yours and you can buy mine. I guess we will be splitting the cost of everything from now on." She laughed. "We'll have an early honeymoon here at Disneyland and the beach. I have my dress and you have your suit. We'll get married at the house with our friends, my mother, your mother and father, and your brother. We'll have it catered and my mother will pay it." They showered, dressed, checked out, and drove to Anaheim.

On the drive, she brought up something she wanted to discuss. "My application and acceptance to UCLA is for Sharon Kelly. If you don't mind, I am going to keep my name, so I don't have to redo everything or make any changes to my identity. Where we're concerned, I will be Misses Cameron, but where I am concerned, I will still be Sharon Kelly."

"I know how you feel about giving up your name and your freedom. I don't need you to take my name and I will never take your freedom. I won't own you when we are married, I will simply be your husband. I love Sharon Kelly. That's who I fell in love with, and she is who I am going to spend my life with."

"I knew you would understand. You know me for who I am, and you accept me for who I am. No one else in my life ever has."

When they arrived, Sharon was so excited she bounded into the lobby of the Disneyland Hotel to be greeted by Goofy. Goofy was happy to see her in her cropped T-shirt and shorts. He hugged her and held on to her until Dave appeared. He released her but still kept his arm around her as he led them to the reception desk. She knew the drill now: she flashed the desk clerk a big smile to make sure he was looking at her and not at Dave while they checked in. The result was a nice room with a view of the park.

She could hardly wait to get to the pool. "Stop lagging and let's go!" As soon as she had her bikini and cover-up on, she took off with Dave chasing after her. On their way they encountered Donald Duck, who like Goofy, was glad to see Sharon in her bikini and cover-up. He gave her a big hug and walked with her to the pool with his arm around her. The pools were crowded, so it took them a while to find chairs with an umbrella. Once they were settled, Dave went to the food window and got beers, sandwiches, and chips for lunch.

Children were everywhere and Sharon watched the chaos as she ate. "What a wonderful place for a family vacation. I would have loved to come here as a kid, but we never took family vacations. In the Winter we went skiing because my father liked to ski. My father took golf vacations in the Summer, to famous golf places, so he could say he played there, and brag about his score. If I ever have children, I can assure you they will come to Disneyland."

Dave choked on his beer. She had sworn she would never bring a child into the world, but she had also sworn she would never get married and now they were going to get married. He swallowed his beer and looked at her as she watched the children playing in and around the pool. She was smiling and enjoying herself.

After she finished her sandwich and beer, she laid back on her lounge chair and closed her eyes to take a nap. She sensed a presence near her, opened her eyes, and a cute chubby little girl of about four was next to her waiting patiently to be acknowledged. "Are you somebody? My sister said anyone as bootiful as you are, has to be somebody."

Sharon sat up, took off her sunglasses and looked at her. "We are all somebody, sweetheart."

"But my sister said you …." The little girl fidgeted with her hands.

"I'm sorry to disappoint you, but I am not a celebrity." Sharon smiled at her.

Sharon lay back down as the little girl skipped away back to her sister to announce proudly. "She's not somebody."

Sharon was dozing when she felt the presence again. She opened her eyes to see the little girl was back. "Will you go swimming with me?"

"Can you swim?"

"I have my wads," the little girl answered and pointed to the water wings on her chubby little arms.

The little girl's mother called her. "Come back here, Katherine and leave her alone."

"It's OK. She is precious. I'll go swimming with you." Sharon got up and Katherine reached up to take her finger. "You are too cute for words. Do you know that?" The little girl nodded, yes. Sharon laughed, picked her up, and walked to the pool holding the little girl in her arms.

She jumped into Sharon's arms from the side of the pool, pretended to swim while she supported her, and stood on her shoulders to jump into the water. She laughed and giggled the whole time, occasionally stopping to put her arms around Sharon's neck, and hug her.

Finally, she got out of the pool and ran to her mother to be toweled off. Sharon walked to Dave, and he wrapped a towel around her, pulled her to him, and kissed her. After the kiss, she took the towel, put her sunglasses on, and without saying anything, lay down with her long hair draped over the back of the lounge chair to dry.

She was lost in her own thoughts when Katherine climbed onto her lap, situated herself carefully, and put her head on Sharon's chest. "Well, hello there. Are you comfortable?" The little girl nodded yes and smiled at Sharon. It was her father who retrieved her. "I am sorry, but she seems to have adopted you. Thanks for taking care of her. Come on Katherine, we need to go now. Say goodbye and let's go. We need to get ready for dinner." She put her arms around Sharon's neck, hugged her, got up, and took her father's finger as they walked away, but she stopped after a few steps, turned and waved to Sharon smiling. Sharon waved back.

"She's the cutest, sweetest thing I have ever seen." Dave had never seen her around children, and he was surprised by her behavior. She rolled onto her side and looked at him lying next to her. The little girl had touched something in her. She had felt a similar nagging months ago at the Chalet with the family there.

Dave looked over at her. "Are you alright?"

She smiled at him. "I have never been better in my life. Will you go swimming with me?"

"I thought you would never ask."

They spent the rest of the afternoon in and out of the pool, and Sharon did some diving, much to the delight of several adolescent boys who watched her intently. Later they went in to clean up for dinner, much to the disappointment of those same young boys. They had dinner at the hotel restaurant with the Disney characters. Several of the princesses were wandering around the tables to the shrieks of little girls who raced up to them to get their autographs in their books. Later, Mickey and Minnie came in to greet everyone and welcome them to the happiest place on earth.

Sharon was having a wonderful time clapping along with the kids. She scooted her chair around next to Dave and he put his arm around her as she watched the antics of the various characters entertaining the children. She put her arms around his neck and whispered, "I don't want to live in Santa Monica. I want to live at the Disneyland Hotel."

After dinner, they went back to their room, watched the fireworks from their window, made love, and went to sleep. Dave woke up with Sharon jumping on the bed yelling. "I want to go to the park! I want to go to the park!" She was bouncing so hard, he had to get out of bed. She had nothing on, which led to him jumping on the bed with her until he could grab her and fall back on the bed with her.

"We don't have time for that. I want to go to the park. I want to ride the rides in the park, not you." She giggled and squirmed in his arms. Dave tried to pin her arms and legs, but it was no use, so he let her up to start bouncing on the bed again. "Let's go to the park! Let's go to the park!" finally she fell back on the bed laughing. He dove onto the bed, pulled her into his arms, and they rolled around in the bed until she escaped. "Let's go to the park, now!"

They were among the first people in line at the Monorail that morning and they rode the last train back that night. They ate al fresco in the park, watched the parade and fireworks, then they danced to the band in Tomorrowland both nights.

The second day they slowed down to take in the shows, ride their favorite rides again, and go to Tom Sawyer's Island. They sat down in the fort on Tom Sawyer's to rest, he put his arm around her, and she put her head on his shoulder. "This is the happiest place on earth. It's the perfect place for our honeymoon. We couldn't have asked for anything more."

Dave thought about Caroline and Ron going to an exclusive resort on Saint Lucia for their honeymoon, Audrey and Jake planning to spend a week at a resort in Mexico, and Connie and Harvin going to France, but all he and Sharon had were three days in Disneyland.

She remained pensive as she gazed out at the park. "I want to wait until Connie and Harvin get back from Europe. I think Caroline and Ron will fly in from New York. Audrey and Jake will be there, Bob and Phil, Sam and Rachael, my mother, your mother, your father, and your brother. Helen can stand up for me and Henry or your brother for you, with Sigrid and Helen's plus-one and us, that's twenty people." Sharon continued, "We'll have a Justice of the Peace do a civil ceremony in the front room and have a catered buffet dinner in the dining room. After the reception we can go to Mother's Blues to dance. I'll call them and reserve a couple of tables. We'll have everything moved before the ceremony, keep what we need for the last week, and stay at my house until we leave. I want to spend our wedding night at the hotel where we went to the New Year's Eve party, in the same room."

"That's it then: we get married and it's Hollywood straight away." He whispered in her ear, "Do you want to do it on Tom Sawyer's Island to consummate our engagement?"

She pushed him away. "Of course not. Sometimes I wonder if you are okay mentally. Do you ever think of anything else? What if a little kid saw us or worse, some kids with their parents?" She stood up and put out her hand. "Come on. This is our last day, and I don't want to waste it, but promise me we will come back here often. We'll be living just up the road."

They got up early, had breakfast, and drove to Newport. He had on his board shorts, and she had her bikini on under her shorts and T-shirt, so they could go straight to the beach. They checked in, left their bags in the room, grabbed some towels, the sunblock, and walked to the beach. They found a good spot and settled in for the day.

They drank beer, ate hot dogs from the beach stand, and joined in a beach volleyball game. They ate seafood that night at a restaurant near the hotel, then went back to the beach to watch the moon on the water. He wanted to make love on the beach, but she told him doing it on the beach was in the same category as skinny dipping in the apartment pool or doing it on Tom Sawyer's Island, it was not going to happen. They lay on the beach watching the elongated reflection of the moon on the water that resembled a giant strand of floating pearls, and the only sound they heard was the crashing of the cascading white foamy breakers slamming onto the beach. They were surrounded by the natural beauty of the Pacific Ocean and watched over by a clear star filled night sky as the earth rotated toward the coming day. He remembered all the nights he had spent on the beach at his grandfather's summer house, but that was on the Gulf of Mexico. This was the Pacific, and he was in Newport California, not a small Southern beach town. It was a different world from the one he grew up in and now a wonderful life awaited him with Sharon in this beautiful, exciting place.

That night, after they made love in the room, she complained of a burning sensation when she went to the bathroom. She said it had been bothering her for the last few days but was really bad now. "You have cystitis. Drink a lot of water and we'll go to a clinic tomorrow morning and get you an antibiotic."

She refused. "No way. I am not spending our last day sitting in a doctor's office. You can write me a script when we get back. You broke me, you can fix me. We are going to spend the day at the beach like we planned, drive to Marina Del Rey, and have a nice romantic dinner. I didn't say anything before because I didn't want to spoil the trip, and I'm certainly not going to spoil the last day."

Dave warned her, "You need an antibiotic, and you shouldn't wait to get one, especially if it's been going on for a while

They left on the morning flight and had just reached cruising altitude when Sharon developed back pain. "Dave, I feel terrible." He thumped her on the back over her kidney and she jumped, then he felt how warm she was. "You have a kidney infection. I told you we needed to go to a clinic and get you an antibiotic." He knew this was a gram-negative infection and gram-negative sepsis was serious; it could lead to gram-negative shock, which was life-threatening.

Three hours later, as they were preparing for descent, the unthinkable happened: the captain announced there were thunderstorms with high-wind shear over the airport and they would have to wait until the weather cleared to land. Dave called the flight attendant and informed her he was a doctor, his fiancée had a serious infection, and they needed to get on the ground as soon as possible. An hour later they were still being held.

"I feel awful. I have never felt this bad in my life." He felt her forehead and she was on fire. He called the flight attendant back and asked to speak to someone from the flight deck. He informed the first officer they needed an ambulance to meet the plane and for the Major Medicine ER at University Hospital to be notified.

The first officer said the weather was clearing but the tower was landing planes low on fuel first. Dave told him this plane had to take priority. The first officer returned to the flight deck and the captain came back to talk to them. "Just touch her. Her temperature must be a hundred and four. We've got to get her to the hospital right away."

The captain returned to the flight deck and announced they would be landing shortly but for all passengers to remain seated until a sick passenger could be removed. It was another hour before they got to the gate. The ambulance crew forwarded her vital signs to the hospital; her temperature was a hundred and five, her BP was 90/50, and her pulse was rapid and weak. She was going into septic shock. An IV and oxygen were started in the ambulance as they drove code three to the hospital.

The ER staff started triple antibiotic therapy, put a Foley catheter in, took urine and blood cultures, and a complete lab panel, before she was rushed to the ICU. The resident told Dave he would admit her to Dr. Sheffield's private service. Dr. Sheffield was a nephrologist.

In the ICU, she took his hand and the last thing she said was, "Hold on to me, Dave. Please hold on to me and don't let me go." Connie appeared and brought him a chair so he could sit at her bedside. "Don't worry, she loves you, and her love for you will pull her through."

The rush to get her to the hospital was over and he caved in. He sat holding her hand with his head resting on her forearm. Her fever was raging, she was shaking uncontrollably, and she was out of it. He knew about gram-negative shock, because he had treated it.

Doctor Sheffield came to her bedside. "As you know, she has pyelo-nephritis with sepsis, and she went into septic shock. She may have suffered end-organ damage, and her labs are not good. I am not going to patronize you, Dave. You know how serious this is, what the survival rate is, and you know the next hours will determine the outcome. I will do everything I can for her and stay at the hospital as long as she is in crisis." Dave knew what that meant. The crisis would be over when her fever broke, or she died. Connie returned. "I am going to stay with her too. I'll stay here as long as she needs me."

He felt a painful intense emotion stab deep into his chest. He had spent a substantial portion of his life becoming a doctor to save lives. Now the woman he loved more than life itself was lying in a hospital bed next to him dying and there was nothing he could do about it. All the years of school, training, work, and sacrifice meant nothing. He had trouble breathing and he was in gut wrenching pain.

He prayed, he bargained, he cajoled, he promised, he called on God, he called on whatever gods there may be, and the forces that govern the universe to please let her live. He doubled over in pain with his head on her forearm, holding her hand, begging her not to die. Dave knew what death was: he had seen too much of it. She would be gone. She would be gone forever, and he would be left alone to spend the rest of his life without her. He would spend the rest of his life as a sad hollowed out shell of himself without her. That thought was too much for him, and he cried silently.

Connie came to his side and put her hands on his shoulders. "She hears you. She won't leave you." A type of numbness set in, and it felt as if he was having a bad dream and could not wake up. *This must be a nightmare: this can't really be happening; it was too horrible to be real. It is a nightmare, I will wake up soon, and everything will be fine.* He sat there numb, holding Sharon's hand with his forehead on her forearm mumbling to her, begging her not to leave him, begging her not to die, for the rest of that evening, night, and into the next day. Connie went without sleep, taking other nurses' shifts so she could stay with her.

On his rounds the next morning, Doctor Sheffield told him there was no change in her status; she was still critical, fighting sepsis, with an unstable blood pressure, and a weak rapid pulse. She continued to drift in and out of consciousness as it went on and on, for another day and night, then for another day and night. Before the dawn of the fourth day, he woke with a start and realized his forehead was cool because her forearm was cool. Her hand felt cold, too. He knew she was gone. He cried out in his pain and anguish.

Many people die in the early morning hours. Dave had always seen the early morning as a new beginning, but for some it was an ending. He lost contact with reality as he spiraled down into a deep dark hole with no bottom and nothing to hold on to as he fell. Overcome with despair, he felt as if he had been torn in half, and half of him was gone with her.

Connie came running when she heard him and turned the overhead light on. "Her monitor is fine, and she is not setting off any alarms!" Dave looked up to see Sharon's incredibly beautiful otherworldly eyes looking back at him over the oxygen mask. He collapsed into Connie's arms, and she held him.

"She is not gone. Her fever broke that's all." Connie held him until he recovered, then checked Sharon's vital signs. "Your BP is 100/70, your pulse is 90, and your temp is 99. Sharon, your fever broke, and you're going to be okay. Dave, she survived. I am going to call the on-call nurse to come in. I need to go home to get some sleep. You should too, she is going to be okay. Her fever broke and she is going to be okay."

Sharon took the oxygen mask off. "How long have I been out of it? The last thing I remember, I was in the ambulance. What about work? Did anyone call my mother?"

"Helen called your supervisor, so everything is fine at work. She had trouble finding your mother's number because she couldn't find your phone, but she finally reached her yesterday, and she is flying in today. Helen and Audrey are going to pick her up at the airport. They'll get your car and the bags, too."

"Did you stay with me the whole time?" Sharon held out her arms.

Connie hugged her. "Yes. Dave and I were with you the whole time. He never left your side, and he never let go of your hand."

"I know. I could feel him. I wasn't aware of anything else, but I could feel him near me. When I felt like I was sinking, I could feel him pulling me back. I know that sounds crazy, but I knew he was here, and I fought to get back to him." Dave was too shattered to say anything. He sat beside her holding her hand until she fell asleep, then he stumbled to the call room and slept until seven. He got up, showered, changed into scrubs, and went back to the ICU. She was awake eating breakfast. The aids had put her in a fresh gown and helped her with her hair, so she looked much better. Dr. Sheffield arrived shortly after Dave.

"Well, young lady, your fever broke, and your white count is down. We will move you to the floor later today. If you stay afebrile on the floor for a day, you can go home on oral antibiotics. Do you have anyone to take care of you other than Dr. Cameron? He needs to get back to his Pedi rotation." Sheffield turned to Dave. "I talked to the chief resident in Pedi. He said you can stay with her until she goes home and start back in the Nursery the following day."

Sharon reached out to Doctor Sheffield. "My mother is coming today. Dr. Sheffield, I can't thank you enough for taking care of me. I am so grateful." She took his hand in both of hers

"That is what we physicians do. We take care of our patients. When you're married to this young doctor, don't forget that when he has to spend nights at the hospital caring for his patients. I will see you tomorrow morning to discharge you, and have you follow up in the clinic. There are a lot of doctors and nurses waiting to see you. Most of them only know you as Baby. I kept hearing, 'How is Baby? Is Baby going to be alright?' from them. They didn't even know your name, but they were here checking on you every day."

Later Nurse Jane appeared with a nurse's aid from Medicine 3. "You don't think we would let anyone else take care of Baby, do you?" she said to Dave as she brushed past him. "Don't worry, we have a nice private room for you. We are going to get you up walking, and let you take a shower. Every nurse on our floor feels she knows you, so we are going to take extra special care of you."

They bustled around her, getting her on the gurney, covering her with a warm blanket, putting pillows under her head, and tucking her in. Nurse Jane put Sharon's stuff on the bottom of the gurney, and they started for Medicine 3 with Dave following behind.

The nurses barely had Sharon in the room before they began showing up: Henry, Harvin, and George first. Harvin and George told her how glad they were that she was okay. Henry choked up as he hugged her. He was completely at a loss for words, unable to express himself as he held her close for some time. He seemed reluctant to let go of her.

Tom came. "Jesus Dave, you look like shit. If I didn't know better, I would think you were the one who had septic shock. Sharon, you are as beautiful as the day I met you. Sepsis seems to agree with you. Are you sure you don't want to dump this panty-waist liberal for a real man like me?" Then Tom grew serious. "I can't tell you how happy I am that you pulled through. I can't imagine a world without you two together."

Richard was with Tom. "My wife and I prayed for you, and we got our whole church to pray for you. You had the power of a lot of prayers supporting you. Dave, Tom is right, you look terrible. You need to go home and get some sleep. Look around you, there are plenty of people here to take care of her. Tom and I will look in on her. You need to go home and take care of yourself."

Jay came. "I've never met you, but I feel like I know you, and I want you to know how glad I'm you're okay."

Jason came with a pretty student nurse. "I'm so relieved you are doing better. I want to meet Lisa. Lisa, this is Sharon."

Lisa took Sharon's hand. "Jason has talked about you and Dave so much. I'm so glad you're going to be fine."

Jason had gone through a metamorphosis that had transformed him not only mentally but physically as well. He no longer slumped but stood up straight with good posture, was well groomed, and it was obvious he was taking pride in his appearance.

Several nurses from the ED and wards came during, before, or after their shifts to say how happy they were that she was doing better. Ella and the ward clerk from the ER came. "I'm Ella and this is Sherika. I know you don't know us, but we know you. I am so glad you're doing better." She had an LP with her. "This is for you. I hope it brings you the joy of the blues to help you recover. It's a John Lee Hooker album."

She tried to hand Sharon the record. "I may not have met you, but I know who you are. Dave told me about both of you, but I can't take this. Dave said your father left you his record collection. I would love to have it, but you keep it. It's part of your father's legacy."

"No, his real legacy to me was my love of music. Please, take the album. Dave said you love John Lee as much as he does."

"Thank you. You are too kind." Their eyes met and the understanding between them needed no words.

In the afternoon, her mother arrived with Audrey, Jake, and Helen. "Your car is safe, your bag is in your room, and we have your bag, Dave." Helen turned to an attractive well-dressed woman with her. "Mrs. Kelly, this is Doctor David Cameron."

She ignored him and rushed to Sharon's bedside. "I have been so worried about you. Helen said you were in critical condition."

Sharon hugged her. "I was, but I am better now thanks to Doctor Sheffield and Connie."

"How did this happen? How did you get so sick?" Her mother was frantic.

Sharon pulled back from her and held her by the shoulders. "It's a long story, but I need to tell you something first. The man you were introduced to, and I are getting married, then we are moving to LA for him to do his residency at UCLA Medical Center and for me to get an MBA at UCLA. Remember, I told you I was dating a doctor at Christmas, well that's him, and we're getting married and moving to California."

Her mother was mortified. "California! You are getting married and moving to California!"

"I know it is a lot to take in. Dave and I were in LA finding a place to live when I got sick. I realize now I should have told you much sooner. I'm going to get my MBA while Dave is doing his Medicine residency, then we are going to live permanently in California. Frankly, I didn't tell you sooner because I didn't want to go through this kind of reaction from you." Sharon searched her mother's face as she held her.

"You are going to move to LA with some man on a whim?" Her mother was incredulous.

"It is not a whim. We have been making plans for our future for some time, and we planned our wedding in the fort on Tom Sawyer's Island at Disneyland before we flew home." Sharon held her mother's gaze as she tried to get through to her.

Helen laughed. "Of course, you did. Where else would you two plan your wedding? Mrs. Kelly, they have been basically living together since they met. They are devoted to each other and the only time they are apart is when Dave is at the hospital or Sharon is flying."

"We are going to have the ceremony when Connie and Harvin get back from Europe. Helen, I want you to be my maid of honor. Audrey, can you and Jake be there?" Sharon released her mother and looked at her friends.

"Of course, Sharon. I am dying for a Coke. How about you, Helen, wouldn't you like a Coke? Jake, come on, I need a Coke. Dave, can you show us where we can get a Coke? Mrs. Kelly, can we bring you anything?" Audrey herded Dave, Jake, and Helen out of the room, leaving Sharon alone with her mother. "Don't worry Dave, let Sharon handle her. We just need to give them some space."

The last thing they heard as they walked out was, "You've been living with him! You planned your own wedding and didn't even tell me you were getting married!"

They met Nurse Jane in the hall. Audrey stopped Jane. "Sharon is with her mother, and they need some time alone, so can you keep everyone out for a while?"

"Trouble in paradise, Dave?" Jane looked at Dave.

"I don't think my future mother-in-law likes me very much." He confided in her.

"Don't take it personally. She doesn't like men." Helen added.

"Leave it to Nurse Jane, what do you and Henry call me?" Jane asked Dave.

Dave admitted, "Nurse Jane Fuzzy Wuzzy."

"Leave it to Nurse Jane Fuzzy Wuzzy." Jane went to Sharon's room with an aide. "It is time for your walk. I will entertain your mother while you do your turns in the hall." She turned to Mrs. Kelly. "I'm Jane, one of Sharon's nurses."

Sharon left with the aide and Jane sat down with Sharon's mother. "You have a wonderful daughter. We all know her as Baby. Do you know he calls her every night when he's at the hospital to check on her and say good night? That is why everyone here in the hospital knows her as Baby. He calls her Baby when he's on the phone with her. Let me tell you a little about him. He not only takes care of his patients, but he takes care of anyone who needs him. He spent the better part of a day finding the ex-husband of a woman dying of cancer so the ex could take care of their children and they wouldn't end up in foster care. He found him and got him to come get the children so the mother could die in peace knowing her children were safe. He faced down a police officer for beating a prisoner in the ED and he faced down another police officer for the way he was treating a young rape victim. He stood up to a drunk, drugged biker who was using a broken bottle as a weapon to threaten the staff. I have been doing this for a long time, I have seen a lot of young doctors come through this station, and he is one of my favorites, not because he is a great doctor, but because he is a good person. You couldn't ask for a better man for your daughter to marry." Jane stood up. "I have to get back to work now, but it was nice meeting you."

Sharon's mother sat alone in the room until Sharon and the aide returned. "That nurse seems to think a lot of…"

"Dave, Mother, his name is David Cameron."

Her mother continued, "She thinks a lot of Dave. I can't say I'm not disappointed. I wanted you to marry well. I wanted you to marry someone with social standing and wealth, someone from a prestigious family with influence. With your looks, you could be the wife of a governor or senator. You could marry someone who could make you a socialite or a celebrity. I wanted to plan a big wedding for you to marry someone significant and important."

"I'm sorry you're disappointed, but I don't want any of those things. When I was critical, yes Mother I almost died, one reason I didn't was because I could feel him. I could feel him there with me. Even though I was out of it, I was aware of him fighting for my life with me and holding on to me to keep me from slipping away." Sharon looked directly into her mother's eyes. "I met a man just like you're describing at Caroline's wedding. He was quite taken with me, and I must admit I felt a connection, a pull toward him, too. I knew I had to be sure I was in love with Dave before I completely committed to him, so I let things develop with this man. I had a good time with him, and I began to think maybe I wasn't in love with Dave. Maybe there was someone else out there for me, someone like … this man." The thoughts cascaded through her mind as she talked to her mother, thoughts about what happened that night at the wedding.

"I never had any sexual fulfillment before Dave. The guy in college was so inept, it was over before I knew it had begun, and with Bar it was all about Bar. I was there for him, for him to use for his gratification. There was nothing in it for me. I needed to find out if what I have with Dave is special or if it could be that way with any real man who knew what … If it was special, was I in love with Dave, or was I in lust with him? I couldn't build a future on lust. I had to find out if there was more to it than that. But that was just another excuse to avoid commitment. Another reason to run away from him. I know now what we had is special. I am in lust with him, but I am also in love with him. I'm sure of that now."

She continued, "I have a problem with commitment. What I did with Alexander was because I was running away from commitment. I was looking for an excuse to avoid any further commitment to Dave. What happened with Alexander made me realize I did love Dave and I want to spend my life with him."

Sharon's mother took Sharon in her arms. "I love you, and I want you to be happy. If he makes you happy, that's all that counts, but I would have liked to help you plan your wedding."

"I'm happier than I have ever been. There wasn't much to plan. We did it in a couple of minutes. I don't want a big wedding. I'm not going to wear white and waste your money on a lavish ceremony. Jesus, mother, like Helen said, we have essentially been living together for a year."

"OK, just tell me when and where: I will show up and wear beige." Her mother smiled.

Helen told Dave about Sharon's mother on their way back to her room. "She sees herself as a Southern aristocrat. I have seen your charming side; you can be a real gentleman when you turn it on. Charm her, play Ashley for her, but don't let her see your Rhett Butler side, I've seen that side of you, too. Save that for Sharon. Did you guys really plan your wedding in the fort on Tom Sawyer's Island?"

"Yes." Dave answered without any elaboration.

"Don't lie to me. Did you do it on Tom Sawyer's Island?" Helen stopped Dave and looked him straight in the eyes.

Dave admitted, "I wanted to, I knew a good place, but Sharon wouldn't do it, so no, we didn't."

Helen laughed at him. "X rated children. Will you two ever grow up? No, don't change. I like you just the way you are."

Jake looked at Dave in disbelief. "Really, you were going to do it on Tom Sawyer's Island? I'll never be able to think of Disneyland the same again. I will be thinking about you two doing it on Tom Sawyer's Island. I'll never be able to get that picture out of my head."

When they returned to Sharon's room, her mother offered Dave her hand. "I am sorry about before. I was so worried about my daughter; I didn't even hear your name."

Dave smiled his most charming "ah shucks, think nothing of it, ma'am" smile, took her hand, and dipped his head. "When Helen introduced me, I couldn't believe you were Sharon's mother. I thought you were her sister. You are too young and beautiful to be her mother, but I see now where she got her looks."

Helen coughed, Audrey hid a smirk, and Sharon rolled her eyes, but her mother beamed. "That nurse told me a little about you, but she didn't tell me you had such nice manners."

Dave continued to smile as he thought, *here it comes, the same questions the gentry in the South always ask when they meet someone new: Who's your daddy? What parish or county are you from?*

"Where did you develop such lovely manners? Did you attend a private school?"

"Yes, I went to a private university."

He was saved by Bob and Phil bursting into the room, rushing to Sharon's bedside, and Phil exclaiming, "We have been so worried about you. You scared the hell out of us. Are you okay, Gorgeous."

"I'm better but I'm as weak as a kitten and feel like s…." Sharon stopped and looked at her mother. "Mother, Bob and Phil. Bob and Phil, my mother."

Like Dave, Phil knew how to deal with upscale Southern women. "My God, you are every bit as gorgeous as your daughter." He took her hand.

Then Bob took her hand. "We are Sharon's neighbors, and she is very dear to us. We were devastated when we heard she was in the hospital in critical condition. We're so relieved she is out of the ICU and doing better."

Nurses, Henry, George, and Harvin kept popping in and out of her room all day then later Sigrid, Sam, and Rachael came, plus Tom and Richard came back, so by dinner Sharon's room was full of people, all of them talking, drinking sodas, and cooing over Sharon. Dave sat on the side of the bed with her holding her hand while her mother got to know their friends. The room was so crowded, the aide couldn't get to Sharon's bed to give her a dinner tray, so she returned with a nurse. The nurse forged a path to Sharon's bed and deposited the tray. "OK, people, she needs to eat, and she needs to rest. It is great she has so many devoted friends, but it is time for everyone who isn't family to leave." The nurse's announcement was followed by hugs and goodbyes.

Helen, Dave, and Sharon's mother remained. "Phil is so nice, but he's a little light in the loafers. All your friends are nice, and Sigrid is so pretty and tall."

"He is gay, mother. He and Bob live together, they're married. So are Samantha and Rachael."

Her mother was astonished. "You mean they're homosexuals?"

"Yes Mother, gay."

"I guess he is light in the loafers. But that sweet, pretty girl Rachael, she is a homosexual too?" Her mother was wide-eyed and shocked.

"Yes, Mother. She and Sam are married too."

"Well, I never. Is everybody in this city gay? Do you have any friends who aren't gay?" Her mother was aghast and pursed her lips. "You're not gay, are you? I mean, I know you sleep with Dave, but you don't sleep with women too, do you?"

"Don't I wish!" came out before Dave could control it.

"No Mother, I don't sleep with women. I only sleep with Dave, and we are going to be married, so calm down."

"Thank goodness." But her mother eyed Dave suspiciously after his comment.

"Mother, he was joking. We love each other. We only sleep with each other. You are overreacting because we have a few gay friends."

"Well, you never know in a city like this where everyone is gay." Her mother looked at them intently.

"We should go and let you get some rest." Helen and Sharon's mother hugged her, said goodnight, and they left.

When they were gone, Dave lay down on the bed beside Sharon and took her in his arms. They held each other until a nurse came in, chased him out of the bed, and turned out the lights. "Time to get some sleep."

The next morning, Dave, Henry, Tom, Richard, Harvin, Jason, George and Jay were gathered in Sharon's room with Jane, Carol, and several other nurses when Doctor Sheffield appeared at the door. "Don't you doctors have patients to round on and don't you nurses have medications to pass?"

His comment was met with a chorus of, "Yes sir," but no one left.

He made his way to Sharon's bedside. "I guess I need to discharge you since you seem to be disrupting the operations of the hospital." A little cheer went up from those in the room. Sheffield looked around and scowled them, "You do know you are in a hospital, don't you?" He looked back at Sharon. "Your labs are normal, your white count is down, you haven't had a fever since before you left the ICU, and there is no evidence of any residual effects from your illness. You will be on oral antibiotics for two weeks. You won't be able to work or return to your normal activities until you are cleared to do so." He took her hand. "I want to congratulate you Miss Kelley on your upcoming wedding to Doctor Cameron."

Sharon held his hand. "Please forgive me. I am so sorry; I want to apologize for keeping you at the hospital and interrupting your schedule."

Sheffield responded, "Don't be silly, my dear. You don't need to apologize. I told you that's what we doctors do. It was a pleasure to take care of someone like you." Dave wondered if Doctor Sheffield was privy to any of the things Mike had said about Sharon.

Doctor Sheffield motioned Dave to follow him as he left. When they were out of the room, Sheffield turned to him. "I'm thankful Sharon survived, and she doesn't seem to have suffered any end organ damage. I have never seen anyone survive sepsis that severe with gram-negative shock. You should be very grateful, and you're an incredibly lucky man, Dave. She is as nice as she is beautiful. The two of you have been given a second chance at a life together, make sure you take full advantage of it." Dave felt relieved.

He waited outside the room until everyone was gone. Carol and Jay came out and kissed each other goodbye before Carol left to go home, and Jay went back to the doctor's station. Sharon was sitting on the side of the bed when he went back in. "I called Helen to come get me and take you back to your apartment. Dave, I can't believe all this happened." He sat down beside her. "I want you with me, I need you with me, but my mother will never tolerate you staying at the house with me. She is just too old fashioned and difficult, but God I don't want to be without you. I know I won't be able to sleep without you beside me."

Helen dropped Sharon and her mother at the house, then drove Dave to his apartment. "You know she will never accept you. You did an excellent job with the Miss Scarlet stuff, but she will still never accept you are sleeping with her daughter. She went through too much with Sharon's father. Maybe if you were Bar and your family had a lot of money and influence it might be different, but you aren't. You're one of the good ones Dave, but I can tell you a lot of men aren't, and Sharon's mother knows that all too well."

She left him in the parking lot and drove away. Dave got the impression from what she said that something had happened with Jackson, and Dave wondered if there was more to it than breaking up with him. Was there something going on between her and Linda now? He unpacked, did his laundry, slept for a while, then showered, shaved, dressed, and drove to Sharon's house. Her mother answered the door. "She's sleeping."

She left Dave standing at the door without asking him in. "Good, I can be there when she wakes up. I promised I would stay with her when I wasn't at the hospital." He walked past her into the house and started up the stairs.

"Don't wake her, she needs her rest." She followed him.

He ignored her and went to Sharon's room where he found her sitting up in bed reading. "I'm so glad you're finally here. I get scared when you're not with me. I'm afraid it will come back, and you won't be with me to take care of me." Dave had dinner with Sharon and her mother, stayed with Sharon until she fell asleep, then drove back to his apartment, and went to bed.

The David Cameron who walked into the Nursery the next morning was not the man he had been. Sharon's near death had galvanized his transition from an immature, naive, idealistic young medical graduate to a grown-up better version of himself. It had taken sleep deprivation, long hours, stress, and the near death of the woman he loved to complete the process, but as he stepped into the Nursery that morning he wasn't looking back; he was looking forward. Looking forward to marrying Sharon, moving to California, completing his residency in Medicine, then living the full, well-lived life he liked to think about. His step was light, and his heart was full because he knew he could face anything now. No amount of pathos, pain, emotional duress, or stress could ever compare with what he had been through with Sharon. He knew he was ready to be a physician, with all that entailed.

After two weeks on oral antibiotics, Sharon was released to go back to work and resume her normal activities. Her mother went home, and they returned to their normal routine as Dave entered the last rotation of his internship.

Sharon made all the arrangements for their wedding. She located a Justice of the Peace to do the ceremony, hired a caterer for the reception, and mailed invitations. She made a reservation at the hotel, asked for the same room they had on New Year's Eve, and made reservations for her mother with the airline. They missed Audrey's wedding because she was still recovering, but Audrey assured her she and Jake would be at hers. Dave called his parents and brother to tell them he was getting married and made reservations for them at a nearby hotel. Sharon called Mother's Blues, reserved two tables, and convinced them to have the house band announce the wedding party.

After she put in for her transfer with the airline, she began dismantling Dave's apartment and her room, packing everything for the movers. They were moving into Sharon's room after the wedding, and carrying what they needed for the wedding, the following week, and the drive to LA in their cars.

The Pedi ER wasn't terribly busy in June, and Dave continued the routine he started while Sharon was recovering; complete his shift, sleep for a few hours before she arrived, go to the pool and swim, listen to music, eat dinner, go to bed, make love, and get up and do it again.

He no longer asked why, lamented about the pathos of the human condition, questioned the presence of a benevolent God, or sought some reason for the horrible things he encountered at the hospital. He simply accepted life for what it was. As far as he was concerned, there are three types of people who exist in the pile of humanity. Those who simply sit on the pile riding it along, others who try to retard it, and those who try to push the pile forward. He resolved to be one of the latter: he would try to help and make sure he did no harm.

He saw abused children for the first time in the Pedi ER, and his compassion for their plight knew no bounds, but his outright hatred of their abusers was even more profound. How sick and depraved was the soul of an individual who would harm an innocent child? Dave dealt with abused women, but they always gave plausible reasons for their injuries, and they were seldom left alone with him by their abuser. When he or the nurse asked them directly if they were abused, as is required by law, most of the time they were too frightened to answer. Many abused women never make it to the ED and if they do, they never report the abuse. What is worse, several women a day, about a thousand a year, are murdered by their abuser.

Men who beat and abuse their wives, usually beat, and abuse their children, too. Dave saw a child in the Pedi ER with a dislocated elbow, a typical nurse maid's elbow caused by jerking the child up by one arm. The father said the child fell on his elbow, which was an obvious lie. He recognized the mother as a woman he had treated in the Surgery ER for a scalp laceration. She told him it was caused by the garage door coming down on her head, but he wondered at the time if the laceration wasn't caused by the woman being hit with something. Now he knew he was right. He contacted Child Protective Services, and they sent an investigator to the ER to evaluate the child. When the investigator arrived to question him, the father lost it, and had to be restrained by the security guards. After the fight between her husband and the security guards, the woman asked for protection for herself and her child, so Dave called Social Services and the police.

Dave had no tolerance for the physical abuse of a woman or a child, but the sexual abuse of either was far worse. His disdain and revulsion for men who forced themselves on women was only exceeded by his hatred for pedophiles, the depraved individuals who prey on children. He saw pedophiles as the embodiment of evil, the most despicable, deplorable, and vile of human creatures. He thought he had seen the worst his gender with the rape cases in the GYN ER until he saw a child in the Pedi ER brought in by a young mother for a rash on her bottom. When Dave took the diaper off, he saw the girl's vulva was covered with venereal warts, condyloma, a sexually transmitted virus. He excused himself, went to the doctor's station, and lost it. He cursed whoever had sexually molested this child to a fiery hell for eternity. The resident was appalled, asked him what was wrong with him, had he lost his mind, and she almost called security on him. When he told her why he was upset, she refused to believe him. "You must be mistaken, Dave. That's impossible."

He told her he had seen venereal warts over and over in GYN Clinic and led her to the exam area. She gasped and put her hand over her mouth when she saw the baby's bottom. Dave and the resident gently explained to the mother that her daughter had been sexually assaulted by someone with an STD. The poor woman collapsed into his arms crying uncontrollably. The resident called the police and Social Services.

The woman told the police she and her husband worked, so she left her daughter with her sister during the day. Her sister was married, but her husband worked and wasn't there when the baby was at her house, but his younger brother was staying with them because he had lost his job. The police obtained a warrant, picked him up, and brought him in to be examined. He had extensive venereal warts on his penis, so he was arrested and charged.

On his GYN rotations, he had seen women with small scars on their arms, their breasts, and even their vulvas. He had no idea what caused them until he saw a child with the same scars and small round burns on his arms. He knew right away the burns were cigarette burns because he had seen them on rape victims. He realized the scars he had seen on the women were healed cigarette burns. This child had the same scars and burns. The mother told him she left her child at a daycare center while she was at work. The police were called, and the owner of the daycare center was arrested. Dave didn't try to intellectualize, understand, or analyze what he saw in the ED. Instead, he had lunch with the Psych resident, and swam more laps at his apartment pool.

Most of the horrendous cases he was involved in were the results of poverty and ignorance. To eliminate the horror, the conditions that produced the horror had to be eliminated. But he knew the privileged would never jeopardize their place on the socioeconomic ladder to help the underprivileged on a scale that was large enough to make a difference. Wealth inequality and the concentration of wealth were not only a part of economic Darwinism, but they were the cornerstone of capitalism. Economic Darwinism was integral in Ann Rand's doctrine of libertarianism that so many in society adhered to as they wholeheartedly embraced the philosophy of nihilism. White privilege played a part, but it wasn't all about race, it was about privilege.

Despite the challenges he faced, Dave was becoming a physician. It was as if he had been walking through a long dark tunnel for the last year and he was emerging into the bright sunlight again. He felt good about himself, he felt good about his work, and his abilities. He was hungry for more knowledge and better skills to help perfect his craft to propel him to better care for his patients. As Connie and Harvin's wedding approached his old understate confidence began to return. Not the cocky swagger he felt on his surgery rotation, but the solid assurance he could meet challenge and overcome them. It was the same confidence he developed in sports. When he stepped onto the field he knew his job, and he knew he could and would do it well.

Connie's and Harvin's wedding was the social event of the season with a guest list that was a veritable who's who. At the reception, some of the titans of business and powerful politicians approached Sharon; introduced themselves, and asked if they could get her more champagne. She was polite as she listened to them talk about themselves and their accomplishments, but when they asked for her number, she excused herself, and maneuvered her way back to Dave. As soon as she escaped one, another swooped in to take his place.

Sigrid also received a lot of unwanted attention from the powerful, privileged men in the room. The tall, pale beautiful woman was like a magnet that drew alpha males in the room to her. Several asked her for her number, but when one asked her to meet him later, she turned on him, "Where is your wife? Is she oblivious? Does she not care?"

After the Champagne reception, there was a gourmet dinner with excellent wine, followed by a lively party, and dancing. When it was over, Connie and Harvin left in a cab for the airport to fly to Paris. Caroline and Ron told Sharon they would be back for her wedding, and they all vowed to meet at Henry's family's ski lodge in January. None of them were in Connie's wedding party because the attendants had been chosen by Harvin's parents for their social status and connections.

During dinner Sigrid took Henry to task. "Harvin's family is wealthy like yours, yes Henry?"

"I thought you knew that." Henry answered offhandedly.

Her eyes flashed at Henry. "Will your family want you to have a wedding like this with the same kind of people?"

Henry became exceedingly interested in what Sigrid was saying. "No."

Sigrid's intelligent eyes bored into Henry. "I would never have a wedding with people like these. I would never marry a man who associated with people like these. When I marry, I will have a traditional Danish wedding with my family, the family of the man I marry, and our friends."

Henry told Dave he discussed marriage with Sigrid that night and she told him she wanted to live the simple life of an academic like her parents, who were both on staff at the university. All she wanted was the opportunity to teach and do research. She was afraid of Henry's family. She thought Henry's ties to his family would drag her into a lifestyle she did not want and where she would not be happy. She hated the overprivileged people at the wedding with their disengaged, narcissistic, superior attitude that mimicked the aristocrats of Europe. She wanted nothing to do with entitled people like them, which meant she wanted nothing to do with Henry's family, so that meant she wanted nothing to do with Henry in a long-term relationship. Sigrid told him she would never put him in the position of having to choose between her and his family, so there was no reason to talk about marriage. Henry was beside himself.

Dave tried to console him. "Sharon didn't want to get married either: now we are going to be married and it was her idea. But Henry, even if she doesn't want to get married, spend your life with her. Sharon and I were going to do that before she decided to marry me."

The week of his wedding Dave was having lunch alone in the cafeteria when Mike walked up with his tray and sat down. "Henry told me you and Sharon were getting married."

"We don't want you at our wedding. You have repeatedly called her a slut. I let it go because I knew you did it out of jealousy, but don't come to my wedding." Dave finished eating.

Mike's face turned red and little beads of sweat broke out on his forehead. "But we're still friends, aren't we?"

Dave looked up and his eyes hardened. "Don't come to my wedding; I would have to throw you out, and I don't want to have to kick your ass on my wedding day." He stood up. "Mike don't think I don't know what you did. You sabotaged any chance I had of doing my residency here. I understand that was because of jealousy too, but you could have ruined my chance of getting a decent residency anywhere. You are a twisted, warped person, and I would beat your ass to a bloody pulp, but I don't want to dirty my hands on you. Stay away from me, stay from Sharon, and stay away from our friends." Dave started to walk away feeling good because he had expressed his emotions appropriately, rather than planting his fist squarely in Mike's face, which is what he wanted to do.

Mike wiped his sweaty forehead with a shaking hand as he watched Dave walk away. He knew Dave was more than capable of doing what he said, so he was worried, but he was also angry. Once again, he had been bested by Dave. "She is a slut. She came on to me one night at her house. She didn't tell you, did she? You really think a woman like her is exclusive to you? What do you think she's doing on the nights you're at the hospital?"

Dave walked back, reached down, grabbed the leg of his chair, jerked the chair out from under him, and sent him sprawling across the floor on his back, then threw the chair clattering against the wall. "Get up." Dave's voice was as hard as granite and his words hung in the air as if they were chiseled in a block of ice. Everyone in the cafeteria stopped what they were doing and looked at him standing over Mike with his feet set, both of his hands in fists.

Mike scooted backwards away from Dave and shouted, "See, I told you, he's crazy. He' not fit to be a doctor. Somebody get security!" At first only one or two of the house officers who knew Dave left, then slowly more and more of the staff began to leave, until eventually everyone in the cafeteria walked out. "Somebody help me!" But no one helped him and the cafeteria was empty.

Dave relaxed his fist. "Look at you. You're pathetic. Get out of here while you still can. I don't want to dirty my hands on you." Mike scrambled to his feet and ran from the cafeteria, pushing his way through the crowd outside the door.

In his embarrassment, it never occurred to him that he had lost a good friend. He was too competitive to understand friendship. In his view of things, he only saw others as rivals he had to beat in some imaginary competition he conducted constantly in order to shore up his feelings of inferiority. No one ever mentioned the incident to Dave and there were no other repercussions, so apparently Mike did not complain or try to report him to anyone. He never saw Mike again.

Sharon and Dave spent their last night at his apartment, and she stayed the next morning to meet the movers, first at his apartment, then at her house. It was a bittersweet moment as she watched the truck drive away from her house. She enjoyed being a flight attendant and living with her friends, but as she watched the truck disappear down the road, she realized that this time of her life was over. She walked back to the house to spend a sad emotional night alone. Dave was at the hospital and both her roommates were on layovers, so she was left alone in the big empty house. She knew he would call to say good night, but she needed him with her to help her deal with her emotions and quell her loneliness. She was mourning the passing of her previous life and she needed him to comfort her in her grief, but tonight he was a doctor. She remembered what Doctor Sheffield said and wondered how many more lonely nights she would spend in the coming years because she was a doctor's wife. It was a long hard night of transition with no one to help her through the metamorphosis, so when he came in the next morning and slid into bed next to her, she clung to him crying quietly on his shoulder.

He didn't have to ask what was wrong because he was dealing with similar feelings. It had all gone by so fast. A year seems like such a long time, but a year goes by in the blink of an eye as an individual rush through their life. He held her, feeling her tears on his shoulder, and reflected on his journey. He wondered if he had been so fixed on completing it, he had failed to appreciate it. Had he been so focused on becoming a doctor, that laser sharp focus had prevented him from fully engaging in the rest of his life? He felt he had skipped over a lot of his life like a stone skipping across the water, never diving down to see what was beneath the surface.

He thought about the ants in the book, The Once and Future King. Merlin turned Arthur into different animals to teach him how to be a good king and to rule well. For the ants, it was all about done or not done. Done was good, not done was bad. He wondered if he had been too much of an ant, living his life for the done and missing out on the doing? Not that he hadn't taken advantage of the activities he enjoyed, trips he took, and events he attended. But even his approach to that had been goal-oriented and endpoint driven; not an in-depth plunge that immersed him in the doing. Had he missed parts of his life because his journey had been too frantic and frenetic? Tolkien said, "All we have to decide is what to do with the time that is given us". *Did I spend too much of the time given me becoming a doctor, instead of living my life?*

He turned Sharon's face up to his and kissed her tears away. She responded by pressing her body against his. They made love with tenderness and care letting their grief and loss pour out of them in the physical act of their union. Afterwards, they fell asleep in each other's arms for the rest of the morning. As he was falling asleep, his last thought was that from now on he was going to experience life to its fullest with the beautiful woman lying beside him. Next week he would pick up his certificate of completion for his internship and apply for a license to practice medicine in California. He would no longer be a skipping stone or ant; he would be a physician, and he would drink fully from the cup of life, delving into its depths as he drank, and he would decide to spend the time that was given to him on a full, well lived life.

He woke up to find Sharon on her side propped up on her elbow looking at him. "What gave you the right to come into my life and change it?" She put her head down on his chest with her arm over him. "I didn't even know you existed a year ago, and now I can't make it through the night without you next to me. You're the one who is always asking what the hell is going on. Well, what the hell is going on? I'm about to marry you and move thousands of miles from my home." She sat up and looked at him. "Who the hell are you?"

He put his arms around her. "Tomorrow you are going to marry me, which makes me the luckiest man in the world. That's who I am, I am the luckiest man in the world."

"That's hard to believe, then we are off to LA for two years, and who knows where after that. I bought something in New York for tomorrow night. Wait until you see it, or more accurately, wait until you see me through it." She rolled on top of him. "I love you, David Cameron. I never thought I could love a man, but I love you."

They got up, showered, dressed, and ate, then left for the airport in separate cars for Sharon to pick up her mother and Dave to meet his parents. He made reservations at the French restaurant for a kind of rehearsal dinner, even though there was no rehearsal, but first Sharon had to meet Dave's parents, they had to meet Sharon's mother, and all of them had to spend the afternoon together. She was so nervous, she changed clothes three times.

He was nervous too, and talked incessantly about her until his mother interrupted him, "David, I'm sure we'll love her." She and her mother were waiting for them in the kitchen, Dave did the introductions, and Sharon offered everyone some wine.

"I want all my grandchildren to look like Sharon." Dave's dad was beaming with pride over his son marrying someone as stunning as Sharon.

Sharon accepted the comment graciously but was determined Dave's parents would see there was more to her than her looks before the afternoon was over. The three parents spent the time telling stories about Dave's and Sharon's childhood and school days. Dave and Sharon spent the time anxiously fidgeting, cringing, and countering the stories; refilling their wine glasses, as they listen to their parents divulge embarrassing things about them, brag about their accomplishments, and tell distorted versions of their early lives.

As she was leaving, Dave's mother hugged Sharon with tears in her eyes and said, "If I had a daughter, I would want her to be just like you. I can't tell you how happy I am that you are marrying my son." His mother did not say if she had a daughter, she would want her to look just like Sharon, but that she would want her to be just like Sharon. That was what Sharon wanted to hear.

"You do have a daughter like me, it's me. I am your daughter now." That caused tears to flow, and Dave's mother hurried out the door with his dad.

"I don't know how your mother had the courage to try for a daughter again after your sister died." Sharon and Dave watched them drive away from the front porch. "She was going to try again after my brother was born. She still wanted a daughter, but my dad was afraid something would go wrong again."

She could not imagine what it would be like to lose a child, much less to have a child with major disabilities, and watch her die a slow, painful death. "I see where you get your looks and your BS. Your father is a very nice-looking man, and he is very charming. You obviously learned that smooth Southern gentleman act from him. Was he a good athlete, too?"

"No, my mother was the athlete. You asked about her courage; I can tell you she is a lot tougher than she looks. She raised two wild boys with an iron hand. If we didn't behave or failed to exhibit proper manners, she would put a major hurt on us, and if we didn't respond, she cracked down on us harder, smiling the whole time. She loved us unconditionally, protected us like a mother lion, encouraging and supporting us in everything we did, but we were raised to be gentlemen, and God help us if we failed to meet her expectations in deportment." He put his arms around her. "I am a mama's boy in case you didn't know. I owe any success I have had in life to my mother."

"I'm glad you love your mother. So many men have problems with women because they had problems with their mother. I love my mother too. She's difficult, but she loved me, supported me, and has always been there for me. It's a shame my father turned out to be such an asshole. She was a lot different before he treated us the way he did. The circus he created around the divorce made her very bitter."

That night they all walked to the restaurant together and when they arrived, Henry told the waiter to bring several bottles of Champagne and put everything on a tab for him. Once they were seated, he had the waiter open the Champagne and when their glasses were full, he stood up. "You are lucky if you have one true friend in your life. I must be lucky, because Dave is a true friend. You are fortunate if you meet exceptional people in your life. I must be fortunate, because I met Sharon and she is an exceptional woman. I'm incredibly happy that my best friend is marrying such an exceptional woman. I knew when I introduced them, they were meant for each other. To my best friend and his exceptional bride."

Helen stood up. "Sharon is my best friend. We went through training together, fly together, and live together. Because I live with her, I see a different side of their love than the one we all saw the night they met. I see how they play with each other. How they make each other happy. I see the passion too, make no mistake about that. You have to be careful not to stand too close or you might get singed, but there is so much more to their love than passion. To Sharon and Dave, to their love."

Dave's dad stood up. "I want to welcome Sharon to our family. What a warm, intelligent woman she is. Of all my son's accomplishments, making her his wife is the one I am most proud of. To my future daughter-in-law, Sharon."

Sharon's mother stood up. "I'm proud of my daughter, too. I'm proud of her courage. She is moving thousands of miles away to start a new life. I couldn't understand why until I saw how Dave never left her side when she was in the hospital and spent every minute he could with her while she recovered at home. I understand now why she is doing what she is doing; it is because of him. To Dave. To the man I know will take care of my daughter."

Dave's mother stood up last. "I want to drink to the future. I want to drink to Sharon's and Dave's future, to their future family, to their children. To my … ah, our Grandchildren" Dave looked at Sharon as they drank. She was smiling back at his mother. He knew his mother was the quintessential mother and she defined herself as a mother, so he was not surprised by her toast, but he was surprised by Sharon's response to it. As he watched his mother and Sharon interact over the toast, he knew he would never risk losing her again for anything, including having a child. Words are powerful and his mother's words had a powerful effect on him, but they didn't change his mind about protecting Sharon. *No pregnancy, no children, no risk! Never again!*

When the toasts were over, more Champagne was poured, dinner was ordered, and they began to talk. Sigrid leaned over to Henry. "This is the way a wedding should be: family and friends eating, drinking, and having an enjoyable time. A simple family affair about love, children, and bringing two families together to start a new family. Do you agree?"

Henry took her hand under the table. "If you marry me, you can have any kind of wedding you want, anywhere you want." That was not what he had intended to say, but he couldn't help himself.

"No Henry, we discussed it, we go on like this. Maybe we will go on like this permanently, maybe not, I don't know. We will see. Many couples in Europe live together and even have children together without being married. Marriage is a legal contract binding two people together. If two people love each other, their love should be all they need to tie them together, and they should not need a contract. I don't want to be legally bound to you and your family."

"Please marry me, Sigrid. You won't be bound to my family. You'll be bound to me." Henry pleaded.

Sigrid made her position clear. "I am already bound to you, Henry. Your family handcuffed me to your bed with golden handcuffs. They funded my research for another year on the condition I stay here. I could not refuse because of the benefit that was to my project, so I prostituted myself. I did it for my research, not for personal gain, so I can live with that. But when that year is over, I am returning to Denmark and my position in Copenhagen. I love you Henry but understand, I will never let you or your family control my life again. I will be in Copenhagen waiting for you. If you genuinely love me and want to have a life dedicated to science and research, come for me there. I told you I would not make you choose between me and your family, but you have to choose between me and your current life, because I will not be a part of that life. I will never let your money dictate how I live, where I live, or who I live with again and I will never marry you."

Henry's face fell, his shoulders sagged, and his usual confident, self-assured manner disappeared in the wake of what Sigrid said. She squeezed his hand. "But we have an entire year together. We have our work, and we have each other for another year here. There is no reason to be sad, and there is no reason to discuss it anymore. Let us be happy and enjoy this time we have together. Let us love, laugh, and live. We have two good friends who are getting married, let us celebrate and rejoice with them."

Pragmatic Henry realized what she said was true and unemotional Henry took control again. "You're right. It's time to celebrate and enjoy our friends' happiness. We'll deal with our situation when the time comes."

After the Champagne, they were an incredibly happy group as they walked back to the house. Before she left, Dave's mother took Sharon aside. "I couldn't ask for a more wonderful daughter-in-law." She whispered in her ear, "Please have a little girl for me. That is all I ask. Have a sweet little baby girl for me." She stepped back and Sharon saw tears overflow from her eyes, then she rushed out with Dave's father so no one would see her cry.

Sharon's mother went upstairs thinking Dave was going back to his apartment, so she was surprised when both Dave and Sharon followed her upstairs to go to Sharon's room. The look she gave them at the top of the stairs was definitely not one of approval.

When they were in her room, Dave took her in his arms, "Do you have one of those little numbers you can put on so I can take it off?"

"I have to undress first, and I have a feeling that once I take my clothes off, we'll never get around to me putting on one of my little numbers." They undressed and she was right, he couldn't wait for her to put a negligee on.

She stopped him. "I can't do it with my mother in the house. I am sorry, not after that look she gave me."

Their wedding day was warm and sunny, not too hot without a cloud in the sky. Dave and Sharon slept late and stayed in bed enjoying the peaceful morning until there was a knock on the door. "It's late and you have a wedding at four. You need to get up and get something to eat."

"Mother!" Sharon sat up. "OK, Mom, we're up. We'll be down in a minute." Sharon tried to get out of bed, but Dave caught her and pulled her back. "I told you no, not with her in the house, and now you want to do it with her right outside the door? You have to wait until we're legal. Now, get up and put something on."

They went downstairs where Helen, Caroline, and Audrey were waiting. "Hurry and get dressed. We are off to the spa for a steam, sauna, and hot tub then hair, nails, and makeup. We'll have lunch, and if you hurry, we will be back in time for your wedding." Helen smiled at Dave. "Slept late, did we?"

"Dave, can I make you a sandwich or a late breakfast? Say goodbye to Sharon; you won't see her again until the wedding." Sharon and her friends ran upstairs to get her ready for her spa day. "I am sorry

I knocked on the door, but the girls were anxious to go, and it was getting late."

"No problem, we were just enjoying the morning. A sandwich will be fine. Thank you." Dave sat down and waited. It wasn't long before Sharon and her friends rushed out the door laughing and shouting, "bye" as they went.

Sharon's mother sat a ham sandwich, chips, and a Coke in front of him. "Sharon said that's what you usually eat if you're not at the hospital." He ate, went upstairs, dressed, and left to pick up Sharon's flowers. When he returned, he went to her room to get ready for the wedding. He had two simple matching bands of gold and Sharon's bouquet of roses with white baby's breath in a plastic bag. Sharon was getting dressed in Helen's room, so he left the larger ring with the bouquet on Helen's bedside table, went back to the bathroom, stripped off his clothes, and took a nice, long, hot soak in the tub.

As he soaked, he experienced a flashback of the past year, followed by a condensed replay of his life. He thought about Dickens' David Copperfield. "Whether I shall turn out to be the hero of my own life or … I am born." He toweled off, went back to her room, and lay on the bed looking up at the ceiling. *Will I turn out to be the hero of my own life?*

He smelled her in the bedding, her essence, her clean freshness, and a heady mixture of the perfumes she wore. He rolled over and buried his face in her pillow, inhaling her and remembering her smell in his bedding after she left his apartment that first night. "God, I love her so much, please never let anything happen to her again," he asked out loud, then he got up and dressed for his wedding.

True to her word, Sharon's mother wore beige and greeted everyone as they arrived. Bob, Phil, Sam, Rachael, Connie, Harvin, Jake, Ron, and Linda, who was Helen's plus one, all gathered in the front room. Caroline, Helen, and Audrey stayed upstairs in Helen's room helping Sharon get ready. Henry and Sigrid arrived with Henry in a new custom-tailored suit and Sigrid in a dress Henry insisted on buying for her for the occasion, then Dave's mother, father, and brother were at the front door. The last to arrive were the Justice of the Peace and the caterer.

The girls filed down from Helen's room one at a time with Helen last. She nodded to everyone then took her place beside the judge at the front of the room. Dave gave Henry the ring and went to the bottom of the stairs to wait for Sharon, as everyone found a seat and Henry took his place beside the judge facing Helen.

She sat on the side of Helen's bed, took some deep breaths, stood up and looked at herself in the mirror one last time, then mentally said goodbye to her old life, opened the door, and walked down the stairs to her new one.

The dress displayed her physical assets in a subtle, yet alluring way, and her makeup had been done by a professional who accentuated her beauty without using an excess of product. The hair stylist had high-lighted the gold accents in her hair and produced small ringlets that framed her face. Around her head was a halo of baby's breath that matched the baby's breath in her bouquet and gave her an innocent, pure look. Her satin pumps matched her dress and accentuated her long slender legs.

"Stand there and let me look at you. I never want to forget how you look today." Then he took her hand, led her to the opening to the front room, and stood for a moment so everyone could see her.

Sharon's appearance produced some murmurs and Dave's brother blurted out, "Damn!" He leaned over to his mother. "You told me she was pretty, but damn!"

The civil ceremony went quickly and ended with Dave and Sharon kissing passionately, as everyone crowded around them. They broke the kiss and looked at each other. "We did it." "Yes, we did."

Helen hugged Sharon. "I am going to miss you."

Henry hugged Dave. "It won't be the same here without you."

Sharon's mother hugged her, then Dave, doing her best to look happy. Her dream wedding for Sharon would have been more like

Connie's wedding. Dave's mother hugged them, telling them how happy she was. Dave's father was smiling as he congratulated the couple, telling Sharon she was the most beautiful bride he had ever seen.

When she met Dave's brother, Sharon did a double take, looking at him, then looking at Dave because he was simply a bigger version of Dave.

He hugged her, then stepped back to look at her. "I only want to know one thing. Do you have a sister?" She told him no; she was an only child. "Damn!" he said, then turned to his brother. "Our cousin was wrong about you. You didn't end up in the barnyard. You landed on the prettiest flower in the garden." He turned back to Sharon. "Welcome to our family." He hugged Sharon again then looked at Dave. "How many times do I get to hug her before I get in trouble?"

She looked at Dave and his brother together. "He looks just like you, only bigger. Why is he talking about a barnyard?"

"But we are very different." Dave didn't answer her question. His brother was a pure athlete. He was drafted by a major league baseball team as a pitcher right out of high school but opted for a college scholarship instead.

"Very different." Dave's brother added, looking at Dave. "Right Big Brother?" He had taken a different path to avoid competing with him on an intellectual level.

Bob and Phil interrupted. "My God, Gorgeous, I must find a new name for you. You are more than gorgeous today." Phil hugged Sharon then Bob hugged Sharon and they both took Dave's hand in turn.

One by one their friends hugged them, congratulated them, and wished them well. After everyone had their time with Sharon and Dave, Henry put one arm around each of them and pulled them to him in a three-person bear hug. "No matter where we are, no matter what happens, no matter how much time passes, I will always hold you two in my heart." He choked up a bit as he kissed Sharon on the cheek.

Rachael took pictures of Sharon, Sharon with Dave, the parents alone, the parents with Sharon and Dave, Henry with Helen, and all of them together. Henry punctuated the whole thing by popping a Champagne cork and yelling, "Come and get it. The glasses are on the dining room table."

Dave's father called for everyone's attention. "My father, Dave's grandfather, is from Louisiana and when it's party time in New Orleans, we say 'bons temps rouler', let good times roll. So, bon temps rouler."

The caterer announced dinner an hour after the ceremony was over. After the caterer's helpers had cleared everything away, Henry stood up. "I want to be the first to introduce you to Doctor and Missis Cameron." When the applause ended, he raised his glass. "To Sharon and Dave, all my best as they start their new life in California." Everyone drank. "This is probably the last time all of us will be together. George is already in New Orleans, Caroline and Ron live in New York now. Audrey and Jake are moving soon, and Connie, Harvin, Sharon, and Dave are off to California. It has been one hell of a year, so one last time, to us."

By the time all the toasts were finished, the wine and Champagne were also finished, so those not going dancing began to say their good-byes. Phil asked Sharon when they were leaving for LA so they could be there to see them off. Dave's brother hugged Sharon looking at Dave. "I thought you were doing an internship. It sounds like you were doing post-graduate work in partying." Then he hugged Sharon again. "Damn!"

Sharon's mother was teary-eyed as she hugged Sharon. "I have so many questions now, but I am afraid of the answers." Then she went upstairs to Audrey's room still trying to absorb what had just happened and to reconcile it with her hopes and dreams for Sharon's future.

Dave's dad was riding high on "that's my boy" pride. "You have it all now, son. You are a doctor, you have a beautiful wife, a great circle of friends, and an incredibly bright future. I couldn't be happier for you or prouder of you."

But Dave's mother was having trouble saying goodbye. She and Sharon had one arm around each other's waist. "I wish I could spend more time with you, and I wish you weren't going to be so far away. Do you think you will ever come back?"

Sharon reassured her. "We are planning to live there permanently, but you can come visit anytime, and we can spend as much time together as you wish."

"I am so glad you married my son." Finally, she hugged Sharon and left with Dave's dad and his brother. His brother went with them because he was in training camp and had an early flight out the next morning.

The front man for Mother's Blues house band announced the wedding party as soon as they arrived. "We are going to take a short break for a special event." The dance floor cleared. "I want everyone to welcome Doctor Cameron and his new wife Sharon Cameron who were just married, and we are going to let them have their first dance alone as husband and wife." Dave walked Sharon to the middle of the dance floor and the band began a bluesy version of Fleetwood Mac's Sentimental Lady.

When the song ended, Harvin went to the band stand and got the front man's attention. As he walked away smiling, a long chord split the air, followed by a familiar riff as the band launched into Chuck Berry's Promised Land. Everyone joined Dave and Sharon on the dance floor as the band tore into the song and Harvin shouted, "We are bound for the Promised Land!"

"Amen!" A black man next to him shouted back and they fist bumped. From then on, any barriers that may have existed between the two racial groups disappeared in the music. The band started rocking, the dancing got hotter, and the dance floor became crowded. Sharon found her groove and let the music take control of her as she and Dave danced the night away celebrating their wedding. Finally, Dave informed their friends that he and Sharon were going to the hotel. "We have a marriage to consummate."

Helen raised an eyebrow. "Your marriage can't get any more consummated. You two have been stead consummating since the night you met." As they crossed the floor to leave, there were cat calls, lewd comments, encouragements to feats of sexual prowess, and cheers with the whole club giving them a loud boisterous send-off.

The hotel clerk greeted them at the front desk. "Doctor Cameron, your room has been paid for and you have been upgraded to the penthouse suite. Here is the card. You will also find a bottle of Champagne and a fruit basket in your room. Here is the card for that. A group of women, here is their card, ordered a wedding breakfast for you in the morning. Simply call room service when you are ready for it. It is a pleasure to have you with us and congratulations." The first card was from Henry, the second was from Harvin and Connie, and the group of women were Audrey, Caroline, and Helen.

The penthouse suite was large, with a living room with a balcony, a bedroom with a king-sized bed, a large bathroom with an oversized Jacuzzi tub, and all the rooms had floor-to-ceiling windows overlooking the city. The Champagne and fruit basket were in the living room and the bed was turned down with two robes laid out on it along with two dark chocolate truffles.

Sharon went to the bathroom with her travel bag. Dave opened the Champagne, took his suit off, put on a robe, and turned on the music system while he waited. She emerged from the bathroom in a long white negligee that was so sheer, it looked like a thin transparent film covering body, and she still had baby's breath in her hair. She walked to one of the large windows in the living room that overlooked the city, just as she had six months before on New Year's Eve. He walked up behind her with two glasses of Champagne, handed her one, and stood beside her with his arm around her as they sipped Champagne looking out over the city.

They understood this was their first night together as spouses, so they took their time to savor it. When the Champagne was finished, she turned to him, put her arms around his neck, jumped up, locked her legs around his waist, and kissed him. He carried her to the bedroom, laid her gently on the bed, and slid in beside her.

He took her to the brink, before moving over her, and she drew a sharp breath as their bodies merged. They rocked together until she moaned, squeezed him with her legs, clutched him as tight as she could with her arms, and they both jerked uncontrollably, merged as one as their passion flowed into each other. When it was over, they lay still and quiet as they returned from the magical place their lovemaking always took them.

"Every time we really get going, I don't think it can get any better, then it does. Maybe it is because we are married now and it's legal." Sharon raised up on her elbow. "It's funny, I never felt guilty when we did it before, but tonight for some reason I felt completely relaxed and uninhibited. I guess there was a hidden element of guilt I didn't know about. I wouldn't doubt it, knowing my mother, and the standards she held me to."

"Let's try out the Jacuzzi." They went to the living room, and he poured two more glasses of Champagne. There were a lot of products in the bathroom, so they added bath oils, bubble bath, and bath salts to the Jacuzzi, turned it on, and got in. The tub was big enough for them to lie side by side as the jets stirred the water making an excess of bubbles and fragrances. After a lot of fondling in the Jacuzzi, they embraced in the act one more time before falling asleep in each other's arms.

The light rode the rays of the morning sun as it came streaming through the big windows to wake them. It was another perfect day, so Dave called room service, and they had their breakfast served on the balcony. They had eggs Benedict, hash browns potatoes, blueberry muffins, coffee, and they added what was left of the Champagne to the orange juice to make mimosas. They ate the chocolate truffles for dessert. After breakfast, they were back in the Jacuzzi, which led to morning sex, followed by another round in the Jacuzzi, then they got dressed, gathered up their things, and checked out.

They returned to the house to find the dining room table covered with gifts from their friends. "I want to spend the afternoon in the park.

We can have a picnic with the fruit basket." Sharon bustled around putting things together to go to the park: a blanket, the fruit basket, a bottle of wine, plates, and utensils.

"Let's go. The park has been a big part of our time together and I want to enjoy it one last time before we leave." They spread the blanket and laid down on their sides propped up on their elbows facing each other with the fruit basket between them. They nibbled fruit, sipped wine, and bathed in the glorious sunshine with the brightly colored flowers, warm green grass, and stately trees acting as a backdrop for their picnic. It was a weekday, so they were alone and the only sounds they heard were the rustling of the leaves in the trees as a gentle wind filtered through them and the far away chirping of some birds.

"I also wanted to come to the park to discuss something with you. I never wanted to get married, but now we're married." She sat up and looked across the park at the houses. "So much has changed." Her mood saddened as she looked at the house that now seemed lonely and forlorn, but once had been so full of life and people, hosting the great parties and the events of the last year. In her heart, she wanted to see Bob and Phil come across from their house with some wine to join them, but she knew they were at their store.

"There is something else that's changed. I told you I didn't want to have children, and you agreed, but now I'm not sure." A small knot of fear started to grow in his core. "In two years, you'll finish your residency. It will take another year for you to find a place and establish your practice before we can buy a house. If we have a child, that's when I would want to have one, after we have a home for the child to grow up in. I had a lot of time to think while I was sick. Knowing I almost died changed some things for me. I realized if I died, there would be nothing left of me, no part of me left in this world. It would be as if I never existed. If I have a child, there will be a part of me in that child, and that part of me will be with a part of you. We will still be together in our child after we're gone." She looked at him, laid back down, and put her head on his chest. "There is something deep inside me that tells me I need to do this."

He was terrified. Putting her at the risk of a pregnancy petrified him with fear. "Jesus Christ Sharon, that scares the hell out of me because of my sister, my mother, and what you just went through. Can we take some time to think about it before we make a decision? Like you said, it will be three years before we have to decide. Can we just be happy and not worry about it until then?"

They spent the rest of the afternoon talking, snacking on fruit, and drinking wine. When they went in, the house felt empty. She knew she could not be happy there any longer. She wanted her own home with Dave. The time of her time there had come and gone, and she needed to move on to her future: a future where she might have a family of her own, in her own home. Dave returned to the hospital to do the few remaining shifts of his Pedi rotation.

Dave was at the hospital, and she was organizing their things to load into their cars for the drive to LA when her phone rang. She was busy and distracted, thought it might be Dave, and answered without looking at the number. His voice turned her to stone. "I'm on my way, and I will be there soon. I can't wait to see you, and I can't wait to resume our life together. Our destiny will be fulfilled and this time we will be together forever." She could not respond. Her heart started to race, she felt like she could not breathe, and it seemed as if a black shade descended over her vision. He had frozen her into granite. "I will come straight to your house, and I can stay there until I find a place to live." That shocked her into regaining her composure and she stopped him from saying anything else. "No! Do not come here! Don't ever call me again!"

He interrupted her, "You don't mean that. Let's talk it out. I'm sure I can make you understand. We are meant to be together. You know that." When she heard him say that, she knew she had to confront him directly. That was the only way to rid herself of him forever. She interrupted him. "No! Hear what I'm saying. I'm through with you. I never want to see you again. Stay away from me! If you come here or try to contact me again, you will regret it!" She hung up and took some deep breaths.

He was parking his car in front of Sharon's house the morning after his next to last shift, when a black BMW convertible skid to a halt in the gravel across the street. A tall lanky man got out and began striding toward her house as if he owned the street and everything on it. Sharon was right, he looked like a rendition of Ichabod Crane. Dave got out of his car and stepped in front of him when he got to the sidewalk in front of her house. "Where do you think you're going?"

"I know where I'm going. Get out of my way. Who the hell are you? Why are you accosting me like this? Move!" Bar tried to barge past him.

"You need to get in your car and drive away right now while you still can." Dave put his hand on Bar's chest to stop him.

"Take your hands off me and get out of my way. Who are you? Is this about Sharon, it is, isn't it? Listen you delusional Neanderthal, I'm here for Sharon, and you need to get out of my way." He tried to push Dave's hand away, but Dave grabbed the front of his shirt in an iron grip and jerked him forward, causing him to lose his balance and stumble.

"I'm Sharon's husband: I know who you are, and I know what you did to her. You're the one who's delusional. The only reason I'm not pounding your face into a mass of red goo right now is because I promised her I wouldn't, but if you don't get in your car, drive away, and never come near her again, I will break that promise." Dave jerked the front of his shirt again causing him to stagger forward.

"Sharon's husband! I don't believe you! You're lying! She's never getting married. If you knew anything about her, you would know that, and do you really expect me to believe she would marry some dullard like you? You're lying to keep me away from her because she told you we're getting back together. Keep assaulting me and you'll regret it. Take your hands off me now, or I'll call the police, and have you arrested.

Now, for the last time, get out of my way." He tried to pull Dave's hand off his shirt, but Dave grabbed his shirt with both hands, spun him around, and slung him toward his car. He landed on his face on the sidewalk and slid along it a short distance.

"Are you crazy!" He struggled to his feet. "You're going to jail for this!" Dave covered the distance between them quickly, hit him the way he hit another player on the field, and slammed him to the ground. There was an audible "thump" when he hit the ground, and "wheezing gush" as the air rushed out of him. He fought for the "wind" that was knocked out of him as Dave positioned himself on his chest pinning him down. He held his ring finger with the simple band of gold on it in front of Bar's eyes a few inches from his face. "I want you to know how it feels to be hit in the face with a fist. I want you to feel what Sharon felt when you hit her. You know it's amazing what the human fist can do to the human face; smash and splinter the nose, cause an orbital blowout fracture, crush the zygomatic arch, dislocate, and fracture the jaw." Bar panicked. He squirmed, bucked, and desperately tried to twist away, but Dave held him down easily using his knees to pin Bar's arms at his side. "I'm not only going to show you how it feels to be hit in the face, but I'm going to bash your face in and permanently rearrange your features." He cocked his right arm with his hand balled into a fist. Bar whimpered and tried to turn his face away. But Dave hesitated. Every fiber of his being wanted to obliterate Bar's ugly face. His arm was coiled tight like a spring ready to explode and his whole body was drawn into a tense bundle of muscle straining to be released. The anger, the jealousy, the hate, the need to exact revenge for what he did to Sharon, all welled up inside him. It was augmented by the built-up stress and duress of the past year. A tidal wave of emotion was ready to drive his coiled fist into Bar's face in an overwhelming psychological release linked to a massive physical action similar to a pile driver beating something into the earth. *This man hit Sharon, this man had sex with Sharon, this man humiliated her in front of her friends, this man abused her. I am going to beat him into dog meat*. He wanted to let the emotion pour out of him through his coiled fist, but it didn't happen, instead it began to slowly seep out of him. *Why am I hesitating?* As he held Bar down, the emotion didn't explode out of the right side of his body into Bar's face, it quietly dissipated, and calmly drifted off into nothing. He dropped his right arm.

Bar had spent his life as one of the privileged few who answers to no one. He had always been sheltered by his family's money and his father's political power. Everyone acquiesced to him and was deferential to him. No one had ever dared to oppose him. He was always in control, manipulating others with his intelligence, and dominating them with his powerful personality. He had never been confronted by anyone he couldn't bend to his will and violence had never been a part of his life. The physicality of an altercation was completely alien to him, and he never imagined a violent act could be perpetrated on him. Suddenly he realized that was exactly what was happening. It was obvious to him that Dave was a man who could impose his will on others physically. That was terrifying to him. An all-encompassing fear griped his body and tore through his mind.

His fear was so strong Dave could smell it on his body. He uncoiled the fist, spread his fingers, and held his hand in front of Bar's face. "That's how close you came." Dave looked at his hand with his fingers spread. "You came that close." He looked back at Bar with hate in his eyes. "Now you know what will happen to you if you ever come near my wife again." Dave released him and stood up. Bar scrambled to his feet, half staggered, half ran to his car. The car threw gravel everywhere until its tires screamed as they hit the pavement and the BMW roared off.

Dave had settled two scores without spilling any blood. He was proud of himself. He had expressed violent emotions without violence. He smiled, *Well, without much violence.* But it wasn't the old "hit the other guys first and hit him harder" approach he had applied in the past. As he watched Bar speed away, it came to him why. *I'm a physician, I don't hurt people, I take care of them, and I do any harm. Violence isn't the answer. I know that. I've seen too much of it in the ER. I can never be a part of it again. That's all behind me.*

He didn't tell Sharon about his encounter with Bar: there was no need to. He was sure he had seen the last of Doctor Bartholomew Augustus Reynolds. He didn't hurt him physically, but he damaged him psychologically. Bar would never forget being in harm's way and how frightened he was.

People like Bar and Mike are everywhere, they can be found in all walks of life, and they never change. They can't. Their personalities are indelibly stamped with finality by their inherent well-constructed paradigms and their embedded rigid, unyielding belief systems. The only way to deal with them is to avoid them. If they can't be avoided, a line has to be drawn in the sand for them, and it has to be made painfully clear to them, if they cross the line, there will be consequences. He had set limits for Bar and for Mike by drawing a line in the sand that was reinforced by a strong dose of fear. Then he left them to choke on that fear while they sheathed and simmered in their own toxic juices. He walked into the house and into her arms content that he had a profound effect on Bar by intimidating him rather than reverting to physical violence. He smiled as he held her in his arms and knew that she was safe.

On his last shift, a child was admitted to the ER with exactly the same defects and deformities his sister had, but they weren't as severe. The child could walk, albeit with difficulty, and talk, again with some impairment, but she was functional, and her cognitive abilities were normal. He had always suspected that mentally his sister was normal and knowing that had affected him deeply as he watched her suffer and die.

The child had gotten into poison oak and had the typical irritating rash on one of her legs. What impressed Dave was how happy and normal the child acted as she interacted with others as if there was nothing wrong with her. What struck him most was her relationship with her mother. It was as if the unconditional, accepting, deep love of a mother for her child had given her the emotional support she needed to deal with others as if she were totally normal. Her mother's love seemed to overcome any physical issues she had and, in a way, healed her of her defects. Seeing how love could heal had a powerful effect on him, and he would never forget the simple case of a child with poison oak. He knew it took hope to carry on in the face of the pathos of the human condition and love generated that hope, but he learned that love could do more than simply provide hope, it can heal.

As he drove to Sharon's house the next morning, he felt a sense of relief, not only because his internship was over, but because he finally understood why it had all been necessary. Like iron is forged, hardened, and hammered into steel, a product that can better perform more difficult tasks, he had also been forged, hardened, and hammered into a better version of himself to become a physician. He was ready to walk among the gods now.

He could not wait to see Sharon, and she was standing by her car with Phil and Bob smiling and waving to him as he arrived. It was time for them to get on the road. The next road. The road that led to their future, a future filled with love and hope.

The author was a hospital chief of staff, a project leader on projects for TPMG (Kaiser) Northern California during the Adult Primary Care Remodel, and participated in physician training as a volunteer at two California medical schools. He has a BS in Biology from Southern Methodist University, an MD Degree from the University of Texas Southwestern Medical School, post graduate training, and was board certified in Family Practice. He lives in Northern California with his wife and has two adult children and a grandchild.

CPSIA information can be obtained
at www.ICGtesting.com
Printed in the USA
LVHW020542080423
743669LV00009B/96

9 781736 759929